Adding Life to Years

Adding Life to Years

Organized Geriatrics Services in Great Britain
and Implications for the United States

WILLIAM HALSEY BARKER, M.D.
Department of Preventive, Family, and Rehabilitation Medicine
The University of Rochester School of Medicine and Dentistry

THE JOHNS HOPKINS UNIVERSITY PRESS
Baltimore and London

The Johns Hopkins University Press
701 West 40th Street, Baltimore, Maryland 21211
The Johns Hopkins Press Ltd., London

The paper used in this publication meets the
minimum requirements of American National Standard
for Information Sciences—Permanence of Paper
for Printed Library Materials, ANSI Z39.48-1984.

Library of Congress Cataloging-in-Publication Data

Barker, William H.
Adding life to years.

(The Johns Hopkins series in contemporary medicine
and public health)
Bibliography: p.
Includes index.
1. Community health services for the aged—Great
Britain—History. 2. Aged—Medical care—Great
Britain—History. 3. Community health services for the
aged—United States—History. 4. Aged—Medical
care—United States—History.   I. Title.   II. Series.
[DNLM: 1. Health Services for the Aged—trends—
Great Britain. 2. Health Services for the Aged—
trends—United States.   WT 30 B255a]
RA564.8.B37   1987   362.1'9897'00941   86-46279
ISBN 0-8018-3455-4 (alk. paper)

To all our elders and
to the special memory of
Mary Randol Barker
(1909–1984)
and
Thomas Reuben Anderson
(1901–1980)

Contents

Figures

Tables

Foreword

There is widespread agreement with the major underlying premise of this book, namely, that chronic diseases now constitute the dominant health problems of Western societies, and that these are concentrated mainly in our rapidly increasing older populations—the "geriatric imperative." People in the United States generally thought they were dealing with this issue, providing for these needs, when the Medicare legislation was passed in 1965, with even a safety net for old (and younger) medically indigent persons added as Medicaid. But, far from having solved our problems, we see them becoming more challenging and more vexing day by day: the costs have spiraled to what seem to be intolerable levels, such that the highest priority for the Secretary of the Department of Health and Human Services is to produce a satisfactory catastrophic insurance program, primarily for older people, incorporating both public and private approaches to payment and addressing both acute and long-term care needs. At the same time that costs have risen we have had increasing criticisms of the quality, adequacy, and continuity of our care for older people, particularly outside the hospital where most chronic care occurs.

With such unresolved issues facing us, we in the United States—professionals, public leaders, and the public at large—should be eager to learn what we can from societies that may have developed geriatric services in ways that can help us. Of such possibilities, the development over the past fifty years of organized geriatric services in Great Britain probably has the most to teach us. This book addresses this need: it provides a thorough, thoughtful review and summary of the evolution and current status of geriatric services in Great Britain, followed by a comparable account of the much shorter and less comprehensive developments in the United States, with closing conclusions and recommendations drawn from these comparisons.

Major themes recur in Dr. Barker's careful review of literature (including official documents) and his own informative visits to twenty geriatric services in the British Isles and surveys of geriatric consultants and general practitioners. These include the importance of a comprehensive system, backed by government; public and professional support, in which there is integration of acute and long-term chronic services; and minimization of acute and other institutional care. Services are organized to meet the needs of all those in a defined community or area. Professionals—physician geriatricians and others—are well prepared through their training to give leadership in providing these services, with emphasis on multidisciplinary participation. At the same time these themes pervade the services in England and Scotland, there is variety as well, described in this book, indicating continuing evolution and further lessons to be learned. Perhaps the most important overall lesson, in my view, is that professional leadership, dating from Dr. Marjory Warren's pioneer efforts beginning in the 1930s, has been accepted by and has worked with evolving governmental approaches to lead to the significant advances that have been made.

In the briefer period of attention to geriatric needs in the United States, some of the same themes and goals have appeared, often learned already from the British: this book describes demonstration projects like ACCESS in Rochester, New York, On Lok in San Francisco, the Veterans Administration geriatric assessment unit in Sepulveda, California, and others; it also describes the currently accelerating development of geriatrics as a specialized field of research, teaching, and practice. But these are just the beginnings in the United States of any coherent, consistent national policy and commitment to meet the health needs of older persons in beneficial and cost-effective ways. Predominantly, as Dr. Barker again documents, care for older persons (as for others) in the United States is fractionated between acute and chronic care, between institutional and community care, and into specialized subsections, each focused on its own high technology. We are certainly still at a stage of development where we can learn from Great Britain, and other countries.

It is also clear that our approaches to geriatric services will be different in certain details from those of Great Britain, given our nations' differences in history, composition, and divisions of responsibilities between public and private resources. This book does not minimize the importance of these differences, but does conclude, quite rightly in my judgment, that despite the differences, strategies and tactics that "have envolved in Great Britain do have exportable features and that these are strongly to be commended to the United States." This book will help us all understand and weigh such possibilities.

T. Franklin Williams, M.D.
Director, National Institute on Aging

Preface

Let us look to America, not in order to make a servile copy of the institu-tions that she has established, but to gain a clearer view of the polity that will be the best for us; . . . let us borrow from her the principles, rather than the details, of her laws.
    —ALEXIS DE TOCQUEVILLE, 1848

Medical men too . . . can doubtless be of some influence in gradually modifying our economic, political, and cultural patterns in America in ways that will be favorable to persons over sixty years of age.
    —LEWELLYS F. BARKER, 1943

Alexis de Tocqueville, the French traveler-scholar, in the preface to his study *Democracy in America,* and Lewellys Barker (my grand-father), in his foreword to Steiglitz's original *Geriatric Medicine,* wrote roughly a century and a continent apart; each offers a charge well suited to the present volume. In de Tocqueville's world, the sov-ereignty of traditional monarchies in Europe was giving way to new forms of government; in our world, the sovereignty of traditional medical institutions is being challenged by new modes of organizing health services (Starr 1982). As one concerned not with government per se, as was de Tocqueville, but with health services, specifically those for the elderly, I share the spirit with which he embarked—to see and learn from the best there is at the time in a changing world. For him, this meant democracy in America; for me, geriatric medi-cine in Great Britain.

The growing demands of aging populations upon traditional health services in the United States and other industralized coun-tries have given rise to widespread efforts to develop innovative ap-proaches to meet these demands. While various components of health services (e.g., hospitals, nursing homes, home care) have tended to respond to demands of the elderly in a piecemeal fashion, what is needed is a comprehensive system that links the component services.

xvii

Since its inception in the mid-twentieth century, geriatric medicine in Great Britain has evolved such a comprehensive system, with a prime objective of preventing unnecessary institutionalization (acute and long term) and maximizing independent living on the part of infirm elderly persons. It has therefore been of particular interest for visitors from the United States and elsewhere to consult the British experience. This volume is an outgrowth of one such inquiry, undertaken in the course of a sabbatical year. My intent was to examine the evolution and current operation of organized geriatrics services in Great Britain and identify aspects of the British experience that might be usefully incorporated into evolving health services for the elderly in the United States.

While the development of a continuum of services, linking acute and chronic care of the elderly in one system in Great Britain, has been critically dependent upon the existence of a single administrative structure—the National Health Service—nonetheless, harkening back to my grandfather's words, it has been the creative work of astute and dedicated "medical men," beginning in fact with a woman, that has influenced patterns of health care in ways favorable to the elderly. The innovative achievements of those in geriatric medicine and general practice, and their colleagues in other medical and medically related fields in Britain, are recounted and analyzed in these pages. The legacy of organizational and professional schism between acute and chronic care sectors of health services in the United States is also reviewed, as are important current trends that would replace this schism with an organized continuum of care for the elderly in this country. In pursuing this latter, seemingly inevitable course of events, I argue that medical professionals, policy makers, and administrators have begun to and would do well to continue to benefit by consulting the British experience.

It is of interest to compare the orientation and conclusion of this study with that of *The Painful Prescription* (Aaron and Schwartz 1984), another recent inquiry into the experience of the British National Health Service in quest of a lesson for the United States. That study focused upon limitations in the availability of certain sophisticated hospital technology in Britain, as compared with American norms, and found the British experience with rationing such resources a bitter pill for the United States to swallow. While accurate in comparing the responses of the two countries to the "technological imperative" that drives modern medicine, the Aaron and Schwartz study has been repeatedly criticized (Kennedy 1984; Miller and Miller 1986) for its inattentiveness to comparative responses of the two health care systems to other important contemporary challenges—

foremost of which is the "geriatric imperative." To paraphrase the situation, drawing on comments of Sir George Godber (1982), the former chief medical officer for the National Health Service, the debate over costly technology, which the United States wins, is about providing "everything for a few," while the debate over geriatric services, which is readily won by Great Britain, is about providing "the most for the most." I hope this book will provide the reader with a faithful account of the latter debate.

Acknowledgments

This book is the result of a voyage of discovery, from one side of the Atlantic Ocean to the other and back several times over several years. The abundant published and unpublished reference materials that were consulted are duly described and documented in chapter 2 and in the bibliography. Less easily conveyed are the generous and invaluable contributions of the many persons who shared with me their time, their thoughts, their knowledge, and their experiences. First among these are my principal mentors in the United States and Great Britain, respectively, T. Franklin Williams, M.D. and James Williamson, C.B.E., both of whom are among the world's foremost clinicians, academicians, and statesmen in the field of geriatric medicine.

Hosts for my formal visits to twenty geriatric medicine units in Great Britain in 1982 and 1983 include, in addition to Professor Williamson and colleagues at the City Hospital, Edinburgh, the following: Dr. James Andrews, West Middlesex Hospital, Isleworth; Professor Tom Arie, Sherwood Hospital, Nottingham; Professor John Brocklehurst, University Hospital of South Manchester; Professor J. Grimley Evans, Newcastle General Hospital, Newcastle-upon-Tyne; Professor Norman Exton-Smith, St. Pancras Hospital, London; Professor Malcolm Hodkinson, Hammersmith Hospital, London; Dr. Peter Horrocks, Kingston General Hospital, Hull; Dr. R. E. Irvine, St. Helen's Hospital, Hastings; Professor Bernard Isaacs, Selly Oak Hospital, Birmingham; Dr. Robin Kennedy, Stobhill General Hospital, Glasgow; Dr. Joan McAlpine, Royal Alexandra Infirmary, Paisley; Professor Peter Millard, St. George's Hospital, London; Dr. T. D. O'Brien, Oldham and District General Hospital, Oldham; Professor John Pathy, University Hospital of Wales, Cardiff; Dr. R. T. Ritchie, Royal Victoria Hospital, Dundee; Dr. Ikram Shah, Maelor General Hospital, Wrexham; Dr. Ivan Walton, Charing Cross Hospital, London; Dr. David Wayne, Northgate Hospital, Great Yarmouth; Dr. Leo Wollner, Radcliffe Infirmary, Oxford.

Other consultants in geriatric medicine whose counsel I should particularly like to acknowledge are Sir Ferguson Anderson, Glasgow; Drs. Colin Currie and Roger Smith, Edinburgh; Dr. Keith Andrews, Manchester; Drs. Patrick Murphy and Michael Whitelaw, London. General practitioners with whom I visited and learned about medical care of the elderly in the community include Drs. William Mathewson, William Patterson, and their practice associates, and Dr. Graham Buckley, Edinburgh; Professor Hamish Barber, Glasgow; and Dr. Campbell Murdoch, Dundee. From the community and social medicine perspective, the views of the following persons with whom I met were most valuable: Sir John Brotherston, Edinburgh; Professor Thomas McKeown, Birmingham; Dr. Muir Gray, Oxford; and Dr. Dierdre Hine, Cardiff.

Many persons working with the various programs of the Lothian Health Board and the Lothian Social Work Department (Edinburgh) contributed to my understanding of the organization of institutional and community services for the elderly, as presented in chapters 4 and 7.

In the United States, I would like to acknowledge my department chairman Robert Berg who provided more than ample time for me to undertake this work; and for their interest and advice related to this book, colleagues Stephen Kunitz and James Zimmer of the Department of Preventive Medicine; Raymond Diehl, Anthony Izzo, Peter Mott, and other colleagues at Monroe Community Hospital; Gerald Eggert and Bruce Friedman of the Monroe County Long-Term Care Program and my friend John Fedoruk, a sensitive and scholarly adviser. Many persons working with government agencies, private foundations, and special projects concerned with the health of the elderly in the United States were most helpful in response to my inquiring letters and telephone calls.

Ms. Wendy Harris, science editor for the Johns Hopkins University Press, Ms. Kathryn Gohl, copy editor, Ms. Therese Boyd, production editor, and many others with the Press have given much valued expertise to the production of the book. Art work for a number of the figures was masterfully executed by Ms. Susan Moran, and Joseph Barker prepared the bibliography with meticulous care. Mrs. Audrey Hogg and Mrs. Helen Weeks provided essential secretarial services in Edinburgh and Rochester, respectively.

At home my wife Malla, daughter Maria, and Scottish lass Shona, provided gentle advice and abundant good cheer under all weather conditions.

Adding Life to Years

CHAPTER 1

The Geriatric Imperative and Organized Health Services

The demographic revolution of the late twentieth and early twenty-first centuries—the unprecedented rise in both the number and proportion of the elderly in the United States—has been repeatedly noted in official documents, professional journals, and the popular press. . . . Perhaps nowhere will the impact be greater than in the health field. The "geriatric imperative" will increasingly influence biomedical research and teaching, as well as the organization and financing of health care, for the next half-century or longer.
—A. R. SOMERS, 1981

The "geriatric imperative" speaks quietly but persistently by way of the well-known demographic trends and high rates of mortality and morbidity associated with old age. It speaks more vociferously when dollars are added. It reaches intolerable dissonance as individuals, families, institutions, and communities increasingly encounter situations such as the following from the annals of a county long-term care ombudsman:

She gets at least one call a week from distraught relatives of an elderly man or woman who either has been denied admission to a hospital or who they feel is being kicked out too soon. One such call came from the son of a woman admitted to a hospital with a broken hip. After a week the hospital was not satisfied with her progress. The hospital tried to get the woman admitted to a second hospital, which has a rehabilitation program. That hospital, however, said that the woman's condition wasn't *bad* enough. The first hospital then tried to find a rehabilitation program in a nursing home. The nursing home said her condition wasn't *good* enough. Having found no place else to put her, the hospital discharged the woman to her home. Because the woman still could not walk up stairs, the hospital tried to arrange for a home health aide. An aide was not available right away, but the woman was discharged anyway. Her son carried her up to her second-floor walk-up apartment. (Wexler 1986, 4)

This account reflects the dilemma of being "sent out into a no-care zone," as portrayed by Sen. John Heinz, former chairman of the Senate Special Committee on Aging (1985), in characterizing the untoward effects of "the new Medicare DRG system" upon Medicare's most vulnerable beneficiaries, the frail elderly. While indeed the *new* hospital reimbursement system does result in hasty discharge of elderly patients, often without arrangements for appropriate posthospital institutional or community care, nonetheless the underlying problem is not new. Rather, this phenomenon portrays in dramatic, contemporary terms the fundamental failings of a health care system in which approaches to acute and chronic components of patient care have evolved on separate and unequal terms. Such has been the legacy of medical education, financing, and practice in the United States throughout the twentieth century, with acute care in the ascendancy and chronic care largely neglected. The challenge to redress this flaw in an era in which chronic disease has become the dominant health problem is a central message of the geriatric imperative in our society and of this book. It is the contention of this book that study of the extensive experience of a kindred society in facing a similar challenge, to wit, the development of comprehensive geriatrics services in Great Britain, has much to offer American policymakers, educators, and practitioners in meeting this challenge.

Demography, Disease, Disability

The needs for organized, comprehensive services for the elderly in the United States are strongly suggested in vital statistics and demographic data and writ larger in more discerning data that describe disease and disability patterns among elderly persons in our society. A brief review of these data helps focus the issue.

Demography

The National Center for Health Statistics (U.S. Dept. of Health and Human Services [DHHS] 1982) recently reported the heartening observation that death rates for men as well as women over age 65 decreased significantly during the 1970s, as graphically depicted in figure 1-1. Importantly, the greatest rate of the resultant increase in longevity among the elderly has occurred among persons over age 80. Population projections for the United States through the first quarter of the twenty-first century show the proportion of the population over age 65 increasing from approximately 11 percent in 1980 to over 18

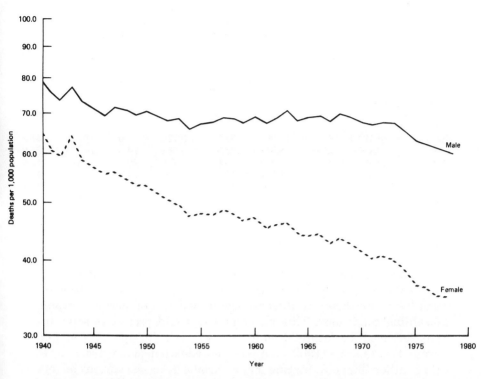

Figure 1-1 Age-adjusted death rates for persons 65 years of age or older, by sex, in the United States, 1940–1978.
Source: U.S. Department of Health and Human Services, National Center for Health Statistics, 1982. Reprinted with permission.

percent by 2030 (Rice and Feldman 1983). Among this markedly increased population of elderly persons, the greatest proportionate increase is projected for those over age 85 (table 1-1).

The recent "discovery" of these demographic developments has given rise to a number of plausible explanations, each of which has different implications for future health service requirements. At one extreme is the Fries (1980) "compression of morbidity" thesis, which argues that occurrence of chronic disease and disability is being postponed or prevented as a result of a variety of risk-reducing and health-promoting measures that have been widely adopted in American society in the past two decades (e.g., reduced smoking, reduced dietary cholesterol, detection and control of high blood pressure, increased exercising, etc.). Under these circumstances, the rate of growth in future chronic care needs would be expected to diminish, relative to current needs. At the other extreme is Gruenberg's (1977) "failure of success" thesis, which argues that prolongation of life

Table 1-1
Projected Distribution of Elderly Persons in the United States,
by Age and Sex, 1980–2025

Age	1980		1990		2000		2025	
	No.	Percent	No.	Percent	No.	Percent	No.	Percent
All 65 years and over	25,545	100%	31,799	100%	35,036	100%	58,636	100%
65–69	8,781	34.4	10,006	31.5	9,110	26.0	18,314	31.2
70–74	6,797	26.6	8,048	25.3	8,583	24.5	14,774	25.2
75–79	4,793	18.8	6,224	19.6	7,242	20.7	11,103	18.9
80–84	2,934	11.5	4,060	12.8	4,565	14.2	6,767	11.5
85+	2,240	8.8	3,461	10.9	5,136	14.7	7,678	13.1
All males	10,302	40.3	12,652	39.8	13,734	39.2	24,210	41.3
All females	15,243	59.7	19,147	60.2	21,302	60.8	34,426	58.7

Note: Numbers are given in thousands
Source: U.S. Department of Commerce, Bureau of the Census 1982.

expectancy among the elderly is largely the result of medical advances, whose effects have been to prolong the average duration of, and hence markedly to increase the prevalence of, certain chronic disabling conditions. This phenomenon would project relative increased need for future chronic care services. Occupying a middle ground is Manton's (1982) delayed time of death model, which asserts that rather than eliminating major chronic diseases, various factors contributing to the severity and ultimately terminal outcome of these diseases have been ameliorated, hence postponing the time at which the individual succumbs to the disease. At the present time, little data exist with which to judge the degree to which these several phenomena and their postulated impact on health care needs have occurred. A vigorous research agenda that deals in part with these issues has recently been launched, targeted particularly to those over age 80 (Suzman and Riley 1985).

Disease and Disability

Chronic diseases and various physical and psychosocial disabilities are well known to increase with age. Less well known, but fundamental to effective provision of health care, is the fact that elderly persons with chronic diseases are two to three times more likely to experience accompanying restrictive physical and/or mental disability, compared with younger persons with the same diseases. This phenomenon is clearly illustrated in National Health Survey data for three common chronic conditions—arthritis, heart disease, and diabetes (table 1-2). As one major consequence of both the greater prevalence of virtually all forms of chronic disease and the greater likelihood of suffering associated disability among elderly persons,

Table 1-2
Prevalence of Selected Chronic Conditions and Associated Functional Disabilities
among Persons Aged 45–64 and 65+

	45–64 Years Old		65+ Years Old	
Condition	Prevalence per 1000	Percent with Disability	Prevalence per 1000	Percent with Disability
Men				
Arthritis	188	3	355	8
Heart disease	132	6	266	13
Diabetes	56	1	74	3
Women				
Arthritis	312	5	504	13
Heart disease	126	4	281	10
Diabetes	60	1	84	3

Source: Adapted from Verbrugge 1984.

annual per capita expenditures on personal health care are as much as three times as great for persons over age 65 compared with those 19 to 64 years of age (Vladek and Furman 1983). Examining morbidity and disability rates among elderly persons in nursing home, hospital, and community settings indicates the magnitude of these complex and costly combinations of chronic disease and disability to be met by health and health-related services.

Nursing Homes

About 5 percent of persons over 65 years of age dwell in nursing homes, and as many as 20 percent of those who are admitted are ultimately able to return to the community; nonetheless, among persons 85 years of age and above 20–25 percent of the population are permanent residents in nursing homes (Johnson and Grant 1985). As the principal health care setting for accommodating elderly persons with advanced degrees of physical, mental, and social dependency, nursing homes reveal the extreme of the toll of the health problems of old age. Thus, the National Nursing Home Survey (U.S. Dept. of Health, Education, and Welfare [DHEW] 1979) found that the following proportions of the institutionalized elderly required partial or complete assistance with the respective activities of daily living: bathing—86 percent; dressing—69 percent; toileting—53 percent; mobility—66 percent; eating—33 percent. Twenty-three percent were dependent in all of these activities. Numerous other local and regional studies of nursing home residents have corroborated this national profile. Virtually all nursing home residents have multiple chronic medical conditions, most commonly cardiovascular disease, musculo-skeletal disease, and dementia. The degree of instability and need for medical care among this population are apparent in the fact that there are about 250 transfers to acute hospitals per 1,000 nursing home beds per year (DHEW 1979).

Hospitals

Twenty-five to 30 percent of all elderly persons experience one or more acute hospitalizations a year, as compared with a rate of about 10 percent for younger adults. While a small percentage of these hospitalizations are followed by discharge to a nursing home, the vast majority of elderly patients return home following hospitalization. Furthermore, the spectrum of surgical procedures and medical diagnoses for which older persons are hospitalized is similar in many ways to the spectrum of reasons for hospitalization among other adults under age 65. However, hospitalized elderly persons differ in one most important respect—their disproportionately high prevalence of functional disabilities. The magnitude of this intuitively apparent fact was estimated by Warshaw et al. (1982) in a series of surveys of patients over 70 years of age in a moderate-size community hospital. Thirty to 40 percent had impairment of either vision or

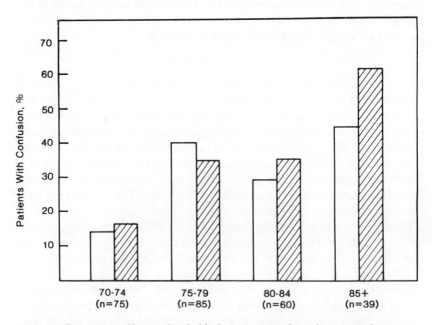

Figure 1-2 Percentage of hospitalized elderly patients moderately to severely confused, by age and sex. Solid bars indicate men; slashed bars indicate women.
Source: Warshaw, G. A.; Moore, J. T.; and Friedman, S. W., et al. 1982. Functional disability in the hospitalized elderly. *Journal of American Medical Association* 248:847–50. Reprinted with permission.

hearing; 21 percent were incontinent of stool or urine; the majority required some assistance with ambulation, dressing, or feeding; and 31 percent were moderately or severely confused. All of these disabilities increased with age, as shown for confusion in figure 1-2. The authors point out that recognizing and addressing such functional disabilities, along with the traditional focus upon pathophysiological disease processes, is often essential to assure best outcomes for patients and to avoid unnecessarily prolonged hospital stays. In another hospital survey, Gillick, Serrell, and Gillick (1982) found that functional symptoms (confusion, not eating, falling, incontinence, etc.) were present in 41 percent of patients over 70 years of age compared with 9 percent of younger patients. The occurrence of iatrogenic illness and accidents was also much more common among elderly patients. The potential relation between these two phenomena, with mismanagement of functional disabilities leading to iatrogenic problems and prolonged hospital stay, is delineated in figure 1-3.

Becoming an "alternate care" or "backup" patient, occupying an acute care hospital bed while awaiting discharge to a nursing home, is an extreme untoward consequence of hospitalization of frail elderly persons (Mamber 1980). This increasingly common and costly dilemma was found to account for 5–10 percent of all medical and surgical bed occupancy in a prevalence survey conducted among a sample of some four hundred U.S. hospitals in 1980 (DHHS 1980). The strong association between functional disability and "backup" in acute hospital beds was repeatedly documented in one-day surveys of

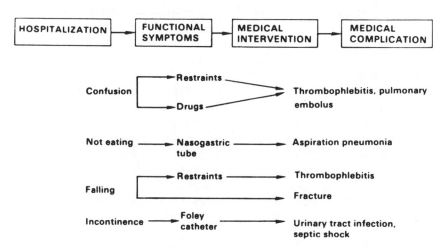

Figure 1-3 Hypothesized pathways for developing complications of hospitalization. *Source:* Gillick, M.; Serrell, N. A.; and Gillick, L. S. 1982. Adverse consequences of hospitalization in the elderly. *Social Science and Medicine* 16:1033–38. Reprinted with permission.

Table 1-3
Functional Disability among Elderly Patients on Alternate Care Status during
Two One-Day Prevalence Surveys among Six General Hospitals, Rochester, New
York, 1982

	13 January		31 March	
Disabilities	No.	Percent	No.	Percent
Total alternate care patients	219		185	
Ambulation, full assistance	147	67	126	68
Dressing, full assistance	158	72	134	72
Bathing, full assistance	185	84	112	61
Urinary incontinence	124	57	110	59

Source: Unpublished Interim Report, Geriatric Consultative Team Project, University of Rochester Center on Aging, October 1982. See also Barker et al. 1985. Reprinted with permission.

elderly patients backed up in acute hospital beds in Rochester, New York, in 1982 (table 1-3).

The Community

Elderly persons living in the community are relatively high utilizers of ambulatory medical services, averaging six or seven physician visits per year compared with four or five for adults below age 65 (Kovar 1983). Furthermore, the majority of visits involve chronic conditions, and these are often accompanied by some degree of impairment in hearing, vision, ambulation, or affective or cognitive functioning (Moore and Fillenbaum 1981). The importance of such impairments is apparent from national cross-sectional surveys showing that the prevalence of need for assistance in daily physical activities and home management is markedly higher with each decade over age 65, in contrast to the 45–64 year-old adult population (table 1-4). These data become the more striking when measured in longitudinal studies of "active life expectancy," the end point of which is loss of independence in activities of daily living (Katz et al. 1983). While loss of independence or death occurs at a rate of 7 percent a year among persons 65–74 years of age, the rate increases to 34 percent per year among those over age 85 (table 1-5). Finally, in spite of the high rate of contact with physicians and the increased predisposition to chronic disease and disability known to occur among the elderly, community-based health screening programs have revealed undiagnosed or inadequately managed medical problems in over 50 percent of the screened elderly (Rubenstein et al. 1986).

Table 1-4
The Need for Assistance among Noninstitutionalized Adults, by Type of Need and
Age, United States, 1979

Type of Need	Rate per 1,000 Persons			
	45–64	65–74	75–84	≥85
Needs help in 1 or more basic physical activities[a]	21	53	114	348
Needs help in 1 or more home management activities[b]	25	57	142	399
Usually stays in bed	7	11	26	51
Has device to control bowel movements or urination	2	5	11	29
Needs help of another person in 1 or more of the above	31	70	160	437

Source: Feller 1983.
[a]Walking, bathing, dressing, eating, using toilet.
[b]Shopping, routine household chores, preparing meals, handling money.

Table 1-5
Life Expectancy in Years, Active Life Expectancy in Years, and Dependent Life
Expectancy in Years, Massachusetts, by Age, 1974

Age Group	Life Expectancy (years)	Active Life Expectancy (years)	Dependent Life Expectancy (years)	Annual percent losing ADL independence or dying
65–69	16.5	10.0	6.5	7
70–74	14.1	8.1	6.0	10
75–79	11.6	6.8	4.8	10
80–84	8.9	4.7	4.2	16
85+	7.3	2.9	4.4	34

Source: Adapted from Katz et al. 1983. Reprinted with permission.

Organized Health Services

From the foregoing data, it is clear that irrespective of setting—
nursing home, hospital, or community—the risk of having one and
frequently more than one chronic medical problem and associated
functional disabilities or impairments is substantial and increases
sharply among the most aged. The data furthermore depict a number
of significant gaps in health services for the elderly as currently
provided in the United States. Among these gaps are the questionable quality of medical care in nursing homes, as manifest by the
high rate of transfers to acute hospital; the failure to meet rehabilitative or other post–acute care needs of substantial numbers of
patients, as manifest by the high rate of occupancy of hospital beds

by patients classed as alternate care, hence persona non grata; and the existence of many unidentified and/or untreated remediable health problems among community-dwelling elderly persons, in spite of abundant availability of traditional physician services. These gaps in health services provision are compounded by the fact that the likelihood of living alone or without family increases with age (Vladek and Furman 1983).

Several important principles for organizing health services appropriate to the needs of elderly persons may be inferred from these and related observations. Given that chronic disease is continuously present and may require medical and medically related care in several different settings, such care needs are most likely to be appropriately and efficiently provided in a system in which services in community, hospital, nursing home, and elsewhere are organizationally linked. Such organizational continuity will in turn be dependent on physicians and colleagues from other disciplines (nursing, social service, rehabilitation) working in collaboration. Furthermore, given the fact that chronic diseases, compounded by social changes related to aging, increase an elderly person's vulnerability to various functional disabilities, it is highly desirable for the medical care system to facilitate provision of "anticipatory" preventive and rehabilitative services for this segment of the population.

In the United States the combination of a strong commitment to research, education, and medical practice related to specific diseases, coupled with health care financing mechanisms favorable to episodic, procedure-intensive care, has led to development of a highly specialized, fragmented, and costly health care system. Specific to the aforementioned needs of the elderly, this system largely lacks linkages between care provided in various settings; favors "reactive" solutions represented by curative and custodial care, with limited attention to preventive and rehabilitative dimensions; and provides little opportunity or inducement for health professionals to consolidate their efforts in dealing with the multifaceted health and health-related problems of the elderly. The historical bases for a health care system so poorly suited to meeting the needs of the elderly are detailed in chapter 9, while current potentials for improvement in the system are discussed in chapter 10.

The British Experience

In a thoughtful essay entitled "Medical Technology and the Needs of Chronic Disease," published over twenty years ago, Forsyth and Logan (1964) examine the challenge to industrialized societies of providing an appropriate continuum of health services for the in-

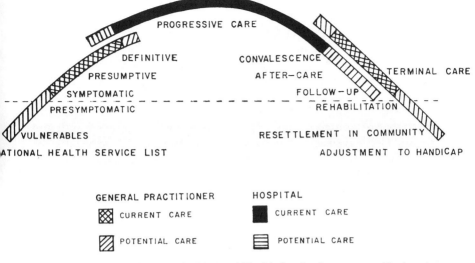

Figure 1-4 Spectrum of care in the National Health Service for persons with chronic disease.
Source: Forsyth, G., and Logan, F. L. 1964. Medical technology and the needs of chronic disease. *Journal of Chronic Disease* 17:789–802. Reprinted with permission.

creasingly prevalent chronic diseases of old age, in the face of increasingly specialized tendencies of modern medicine.* The authors focus specifically on the potential for achieving such ends within the publicly owned and operated British National Health Service (NHS), with its commitment to provide comprehensive medical care for all. Figure 1-4 illustrates the organized spectrum of services that could in theory be provided by the NHS. This spectrum would include preventive surveillance of high-risk elderly persons ("vulnerables") under the care of a general practitioner in the community; hospitalization when needed under a specialist's care, including convalescent and rehabilitative care to complement traditional medical and surgical care; and resettlement in the community at highest level of independent functioning, again under the care of the general practitioner, in concert with various community-based support services. At the time this essay was written, the authors concluded that some but not all components of their proposed spectrum of care were operating in the various parts of Great Britain they studied. Of particular concern were the gaps in provision for preventive surveillance of vulnerables in the community and for inpatient and posthospital

---

*Interestingly, at the time of this essay the proportion of the British population over age 65 (11.7 percent) in 1960 was essentially the same as found in the United States twenty years later (11.3 percent).

attention to rehabilitative and resettlement needs of those with chronic conditions.

In the ensuing twenty-plus years since this essay was written, a process of steady growth and development of the theorized continuum of services for the elderly has occurred in Great Britain. This process, which actually began several decades earlier in the inhospitable environs of former Poor Law institutions, has involved major innovative developments in both the general hospital and community settings, very much in line with the needs identified by Forsyth and Logan. Critical to stimulating and facilitating such innovations has been the existence of a comprehensive health care system, operating under a fixed budget, which is conducive to the integration of acute and chronic care services. However, as discussed and illustrated at length in chapters 3 through 8, organizational innovations in health care evolved not simply from a grand design or official national policy, but from the pragmatic efforts and creativity of members of the medical, nursing, social work, and other health professionals, along with local health and social service administrators. Foremost among these has been the strong and sustained British geriatric medicine movement, which, having begun with fewer than ten members in the early 1950s, numbered over five hundred consultant specialists working in hospital-based geriatric units throughout the country by 1985.

Adding Life to Years, the motto of the British Geriatrics Society, bespeaks the origins and essence of this field of medicine. Of the many attainments of the British geriatric medicine movement, most essential to the fabric of health services in Britain has been its strong emphasis on incorporating rehabilitation and a community orientation into the mainstream of acute and chronic institutional care of frail elderly persons. This approach is epitomized in the work of Dr. Marjory Warren, acknowledged founder of the field, who, as medical supervisor of a large chronic care institution in the 1930s and 1940s, uncovered among her patients many neglected but remediable medical and physical problems that had been attributed to the intractable consequences of aging (Warren 1946).

The recognition that the disabilities and the acute and chronic health problems of old age require special assessment, and are in turn amenable to rehabilitative and therapeutic intervention, has since become the conceptual basis for the field of geriatric medicine. Figure 1-5, from an essay by Dr. James Williamson (1984) entitled "Health Care of the Elderly: Theory and Practice," neatly portrays the relationship between age and the capacity of the individual to function independently, as reviewed in tabular numerical form earlier in this chapter. It is at the point of significantly reduced reserves—the "zone of geriatric medicine"—that availability of appro-

Function in relation to Age & Disease

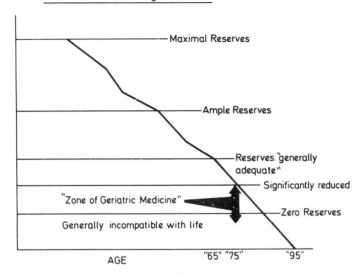

Figure 1-5 The "zone" of geriatric medicine.
Source: Williamson, J. 1984. Health care of the elderly: Theory and practice. The Nova Scotia Medical Bulletin 103–8. Reprinted with permission.

priately organized health services has played a critical role in Great Britain, a fitting foil to the aforementioned "no-care zone" in the United States.

Summary

The geriatric imperative to develop an organized continuum of health care in the United States is manifest by extensive evidence of health care needs of elderly persons for which services are often unavailable, poorly coordinated, or unnecessarily costly. This situation is the legacy of a health care system in which services for acute and chronic health problems evolved separately, with medical education, financing, and practice patterns focusing almost exclusively upon the former. Over the past several decades similar circumstances have been met in Great Britain by the evolution of comprehensive, integrated services for the elderly, central to which has been the geriatric medicine movement. Analysis of the history and current operations of organized geriatrics services in Great Britain and the applicability of this experience to the development of comprehensive health services for the elderly in the United States constitutes the body of this book.

CHAPTER 2

Sources and Methods of Study

The "organization" of medical services in a society is the result of a variety of planned and unplanned forces at work over time. These forces include the cultural, historic, economic, and political legacy of the society; the mechanisms for financing health and social services; the demography and health status of the populace, as measured by vital statistics and morbidity indexes; the state of medical knowledge and availability of resources for its application; and the initiative of individual professionals and professional groups in shaping these applications. The development and current functioning of organized geriatrics services in Great Britain are no exception to this process. The study of this experience with a view to assessing its implications for current developments in the United States was therefore approached as a multifaceted empirical inquiry. Information was assembled through a variety of formal and informal means, including extensive review of published and unpublished documents, direct observation of the functioning of geriatric and related health services in a number of settings, conduct of numerous interviews and several formal surveys, and participation in postgraduate courses and conferences. An analogous but more limited review of the development of health services for the elderly in the United States was also conducted. This chapter describes these various avenues of inquiry and their pertinence to the following chapters.

Literature Review

While much has been written about health and related problems of old age and the various services provided in Britain, both before and since the geriatric medicine movement, no single comprehensive source of this information exists. Therefore, to gain insight into the historical background of the geriatrics movement and the current state of its development, I consulted a wide selection of books, journal articles, government documents, and unpublished documents.

The most important of these sources have been briefly described in an annotated bibliography (Barker 1984). The collections and/or professional staff at the following locations were instrumental in identifying and making accessible these source materials:

University of Edinburgh
  Department of Geriatric Medicine (research and teaching files)
  Department of Community Medicine (health services files and library of the Usher Institute)
  Erskine Medical Library (journals, books, special collection of government health policy documents)

King Edward's Fund College, London (library and extensive files on the British National Health Service)

British Geriatrics Society, London (archives on history and leaders of the geriatrics movement; bibliography of the members' publications)

Chapter 3, "From Poorhouse Infirmary to District General Hospital," is a synthesis of the essential influences and events that led to the evolution of health care for the aged in Great Britain. Clearly emerging from this historical account is the central role of hospital-based departments (or units) as the organizing principle of modern geriatric medicine in Britain. Furthermore, as discussed in chapter 3, three distinctive models for organizing hospital-based geriatrics services have evolved: selective referral, age related, and integrated.

Observation of Services

An in-depth participant-observer study of one geriatric medicine unit and brief site visits to a selection of other units were undertaken to gain clear insight into the practice of modern geriatric medicine in Great Britain. My status as visiting fellow in the Department of Geriatric Medicine of the University of Edinburgh during the academic year of 1982–83 afforded me a unique opportunity to observe and discuss at length the many clinical, administrative, and academic aspects of geriatric medicine in one setting. This experience included participation in all regularly scheduled clinical and administrative activities within the department as well as involvement in geriatric consultations elsewhere in the community. These activities in turn provided numerous occasions for informal inquiry about organizational linkages between the various health professionals and health care settings that comprised the geriatrics service. In addition, meetings and field trips to learn about related health and social services in the Edinburgh vicinity helped me understand the geri-

atric medicine unit in the larger context in which it serves. From
these observations emerged the portrait of "A Model Geriatric Medicine Unit in Edinburgh," contained in chapter 4.

Site Visits

Site visits to geriatrics departments elsewhere in Great Britain in
the spring of 1983, under the sponsorship of a World Health Organization travel-study fellowship, were planned with a view to learning
how the components of the basic model as depicted in the literature of
geriatric medicine and observed in Edinburgh were (or were not)
addressed in various other settings. Selection of sites was influenced
by a desire to observe examples of each of the three organizational
models mentioned earlier; to see examples based in both university
teaching hospitals and district general hospitals; and finally, to see
settings in which there was either formal or anecdotal evidence that
the geriatrics service had made significant impact in expediting
hospital care of the elderly. Given approximately two months to
make visits of one to two days each, I decided to select fifteen to
twenty sites. These selections were made after reviewing the recent
geriatrics literature and discussing the sites with a number of members of the British Geriatrics Society and with staff at the Department of Health and Social Security headquarters in London. A total
of twenty units were ultimately included in the survey. (Fig. 5-1 is a
map of the places visited.) A breakdown of the sites by organizational
model and academic status is shown here:

Models	Teaching	Nonteaching
Selective referral	9	3
Age-related	1	4
Integrated	2	1

A set of questions to be used during site visits was developed and
sent to the hosts at each site prior to the visit. The questions focused
on the following topics: (1) history and evolution of the unit, (2)
current internal structure and operations, (3) relationships with
other acute hospital services, and (4) measures of impact of the geriatrics service on hospital utilization.

The extensive observations from these visits are summarized and
synthesized in chapters 5 and 6. While the details of each unit's
evolution and operation are varied, nonetheless, these observations
reveal a remarkable degree of similarity among units with respect to
the essential resources, professional staffing and, above all, commitment to providing a continuum of services for the vulnerable elderly
patient.

Surveys

Outside the immediate purview of the geriatrics service unit, but also essential to an understanding of the operation of organized geriatrics services in Great Britain, are two other important subjects, which were studied through a combination of literature review and special surveys. The first of these is community-based primary care and social support services for the elderly; the second is education and training in geriatric medicine.

Virtually all residents of Great Britain are enrolled with a general practice, which serves as their primary point of access to medical and medically related health services. I was interested to study both the array of problems the elderly present to the general practitioner and the ways in which general practices are organized to deal with these problems. In addition to reviewing the published literature on the subject, I conducted two special surveys in Edinburgh. The first of these, a study of the "ecology of primary medical care of the elderly," consists of a retrospective review of medical and nursing records for a representative sample of elderly patients enrolled in one general practice in Edinburgh. The second consists of a mail survey of a representative sample of all general practices in the Edinburgh area to determine staffing patterns and special arrangements for meeting health care needs of elderly patients. (A copy of the mail survey instrument with brief explanatory notes is contained in Appendix A.) Chapter 7 discusses the findings of these surveys and relates them to the recent policy emphasis on caring for the elderly in the community in Britain. A limited review of the development and current status of community-based social services is also included in this chapter.

Training future physicians for both general and specialist roles in care of the elderly has been integral to the development of comprehensive geriatrics services. A number of published and unpublished surveys of medical school curricula and distribution of medical personnel by specialty were available for assessing the status of education and training in geriatrics. Additionally, I conducted a special survey of recently appointed consultants in geriatric medicine. This survey focused upon factors in the decision to pursue a career in geriatrics, training experiences, and current patterns of professional work as a consultant in the specialty. Chapter 8 discusses the findings of these several surveys on education and training.

Postgraduate Courses

Participating in three postgraduate courses provided me with insights into the content and organization of geriatric medicine in Great Britain and proved helpful in synthesizing what I learned from the literature review and the various aforementioned observational studies. The courses are as follows:

1. *The Aging of Populations: Clinical Care of the Elderly.* A succinct expert review of all major disease and disability of particular significance among the elderly and the organization of services to deal with them (organized by the Department of Geriatric Medicine, University of Edinburgh, under sponsorship of the British Council).

2. *Management Skills in Geriatric Medicine.* A seminar and workshop focused upon managerial roles the geriatrician is expected to play within the hospital, local community, and health services at large in making effective and efficient use of resources (organized and sponsored by the King Edward's Fund College, London).

3. *Rehabilitation of the Elderly.* A review and demonstration of the special skills, equipment, and underlying pathophysiology to which remedial services (physical therapy, occupational therapy, etc.) are directed in restoring and preserving function in frail elderly persons (organized by Dr. Keith Andrews under sponsorship of the University of Manchester Department of Geriatric Medicine).

U.S. Sources

Perspectives and documentary history on the long-standing division between acute and chronic care services for the elderly in the United States, culminating with the enactment of the 1965 Medicare and Medicaid legislation, were obtained principally from the following books: *Beyond Sixty-five: The Dilemma of Old Age in America's Past* (Haber 1983); *The American Health Care System: Its Genesis and Trajectory* (Freymann 1980); *The Social Transformation of American Medicine* (Starr 1982); *The Politics of Medicare* (Marmor 1973); and *Unloving Care* (Vladek 1980). These volumes were supplemented by consulting a variety of special monographs and other published and unpublished documents cited in chapter 9.

Information and insights bearing upon the rapidly evolving interest in reforming health services for the elderly in the United States during the present decade came from a number of sources. These include regular attendance at meetings and consultation with leaders of the American Geriatrics Society, the Gerontological Society of America, and the Gerontological Health Section of the American Public Health Association; extensive reading in the journals of these organizations as well as in many others containing articles related to health and social services for the elderly; correspondence and direct communication with parties involved with health policy for the elderly in the Health Care Financing Administration (HCFA), the National Center for Health Services Research, the National Institute on Aging, Senate and House legislative committees concerned with aging, the Congressional Budget Office, the American Hospital Association, the Robert Wood Johnson Foundation, and others. Attendance at the following three short courses in 1985 was helpful to me in reviewing current trends in organization, financing, and medical practices with respect to the elderly: "Management Strategies from the National Experience with DRGs and RUGs" (sponsored by the Western New York Geriatric Education Center, Buffalo, New York); "Coordinated Care for the Elderly" (sponsored by the American Hospital Association and the Society for Social Work Directors, Boston, Massachusetts); and "Geriatric Medicine 1985" (sponsored by the Division on Aging, Harvard Medical School).

The aforementioned secondary sources have been complemented by my direct involvement with a number of major geriatric health service delivery initiatives in Rochester, New York, a community with a distinguished legacy of innovation in care of the elderly. This involvement includes serving as an attending physician and consultant in health services research and development at Monroe Community Hospital, a large chronic care facility with a long-standing academic affiliation with the University of Rochester Medical Center; membership on the professional advisory committee for the Monroe County Long-Term Care Program (ACCESS), one of the nation's first and best known community-based alternative long-term care projects; formal and informal consultation on development and evaluation of special geriatric inpatient units in several general hospitals in Rochester; and consultant to Blue Cross–Blue Shield of greater Rochester to study development and operation of an affiliated HMO-Medicare program under an applied policy fellowship awarded by the Gerontological Society of America.

For the final chapter, drawing implications for the United States from the British experience, the following related publications were particularly helpful: *Old, Alone, and Neglected: Care of the Aged in Scotland and the United States* (Kayser-Jones, 1981), a volume principally concerned with a comparative study of long-term institutional care in the two societies; *Geriatric Medicine in the United States and Great Britain* (Carboni 1982), a comparative study of the development (or nondevelopment) of the specialty of geriatric medicine in the two countries; *International Perspectives on Long-Term Care* (Reif and Trager 1985), a volume principally concerned with comparative developments in home care services among several countries, including Great Britain and the United States.

CHAPTER 3

The British Geriatric Medicine Movement
From Poorhouse Infirmary to District General Hospital

*The busy, productive, rehabilitation unit she and her staff had created
within the former apathetic, chronic wards became widely recognized as
the pioneer centre of medical care for the elderly in these Islands.*
—G. F. ADAMS, 1961

Care for the dependent elderly and other vulnerable members of
society in Great Britain became primarily a concern of government
in the sixteenth century, following the widespread destruction of
traditional religious institutions, including charitable shelters, during the reign of Henry VIII. The passage of the Poor Relief Act of
1601, the nation's original Poor Law, formally conferred upon local
governments the responsibility of providing for their indigent and
dependent members. This led to the establishment of Poor Law institutions (poorhouses, workhouses) as the largely exclusive source of
"relief" for young and old alike who were unable to provide for themselves (Schweinitz 1961). As numbers of elderly with chronic disability and disease in these institutions increased in the nineteenth
century, infirmaries were developed. These Poor Law institutions
were administered by local Boards of Guardians, which generally
sought to maintain the inmates at minimal public expense. Little if
any medical care was provided. This pattern of public institutional
care for dependent elderly persons evolved parallel with the development of voluntary general and specialty hospitals, which defined
their task as the provision of short-term acute medical and surgical
care. Physicians and surgeons, forerunners of the hospital consultant specialist, regularly treated patients and taught medical students in these settings. Mounting pressure, in the later part of the
nineteenth century, for the voluntary hospitals to admit chronically
ill elderly persons who might block beds was met by official policies,
first propagated by St. Thomas's Hospital in London, to exclude such

patients from their wards. Physicians and surgeons confined their hospital work, including teaching medical students, almost exclusively to the voluntary institutions (Abel-Smith 1964; Townsend 1962).

Toward the end of the nineteenth century, county and municipal infectious disease hospitals began to appear as part of the public health movement to contain epidemic disease. Metropolitan Asylum Boards with a medical orientation (effectively local hospital administrations) were created to oversee these public hospitals, and staff physicians as well as consultants from the voluntary hospitals were engaged to provide medical care. While of no direct benefit to the institutionalized elderly, this third aspect of hospital development represented a significant advance with future applicability to the care of the elderly: public hospitals with full-time medical staffing (Abel-Smith 1964, ch. 8).

Developments in the Early Twentieth Century

Professional, institutional, and administrative separation between acute and chronic care persisted well into the twentieth century. However, several developments in the 1930s and 1940s laid the ground for change. The Local Government Act of 1929, the culmination of many years of parliamentary effort to reform the archaic Poor Laws of past centuries, provided local government with authority and financial incentives to transfer the administration of Poor Law infirmaries to the public health and hospital sector alongside the municipal infectious disease hospitals. Some localities responded vigorously in transforming infirmaries to public chronic care hospitals; however, in many instances entrenched Poor Law guardians thwarted change and retained the infirmaries in their traditional miserly, nontherapeutic mode (Abel-Smith 1964, chs. 22 and 23).

Among the progressive counties, West Middlesex, adjacent to London, stands out. The county public hospital administration assumed responsibility for a large local poorhouse infirmary occupied by approximately seven hundred bedridden, chronically ill, mostly elderly patients and recruited medical staff from the nearby West Middlesex (teaching) Hospital. Dr. Marjory Warren, a surgeon by training, assumed the post of deputy medical director in the early 1930s and in the succeeding decade revolutionized the process of patient care by applying techniques that have become the hallmark of geriatric medicine in Great Britain. In essence this consisted of a multidisciplinary assessment and rehabilitation approach to the infirm elderly, relegating such patients to permanent institutionalization only as a last resort. As an early result of this active approach, some 200 of the original 700 chronically ill elderly were restored sufficiently to independent function that they were discharged to residential accommodations. Previously, virtually all such patients had remained institutionalized and bedridden until death (Warren 1948). Reflecting on how this approach might optimally develop throughout the country, Dr. Warren articulated many essential ingredients, including the creation of a medical specialty of geriatrics, the importance of multidisciplinary assessment, and the placing of geriatric medicine units in general hospitals. She furthermore emphasized that such a strategy should yield a significant reduction in the problem of bed blocking by chronically ill patients (Warren 1946). Her many accomplishments and publications are succinctly reviewed in a recent article by Matthews (1984).

With the outbreak of World War II, the British Ministry of Health created an Emergency Medical Service, primarily to assure ample hospital beds to care for anticipated civilian casualties. While inventorying the nation's hospitals, the ministry became aware for the first time of the massive numbers of disabled elderly persons in public hospitals. Most were receiving only custodial care, in contrast to the exceptional services developed at a few sites such as the West Middlesex County Hospital. The imperative to address medical needs of this class of patients, both for their own benefit and for the benefit of present and future hospital services of Great Britain, was recorded by the ministry (Townsend 1962).

The National Health Service Act, legislated in 1946 and implemented in 1948, conferred upon the Ministry of Health the duty of promoting "a free comprehensive health service designed to secure improvement in the physical and mental health of the people" (Great Britain, National Health Service 1946, 123).* The principal achievement of the act insofar as the evolution of health service for the frail elderly was concerned was to transfer ownership of all public and voluntary hospitals to the Ministry of Health. With this action came the commitment to provide consultant-level medical care to patients with long-term chronic illness as well as to those with short-term acute illness (Abel-Smith 1964, ch. 29). In addressing this issue, Dr. E. L. Sturdee, a senior medical officer in the ministry responsible for medical aspects of former Poor Law institutions, became aware of Dr. Warren's accomplishments in West Middlesex. Sturdee and a medical colleague in Parliament, Lord Amulree, worked through their official positions to bring this experience to the attention of government and professional groups (Sheldon 1971; Adams 1975).

*A good general account of the origins and operations of the British National Health Services is contained in Pater 1981.

In response to such stimuli, varying developments anticipated the emergence of the network of district-based geriatric services that now exist throughout Great Britain. In 1947 Warren, Amulree, and other "pioneers" of geriatric medicine formed the British Geriatrics Society (BGS) to promote improved standards of medical services for the elderly sick (Howell 1974). The British Medical Association (BMA) appointed a committee, including several original members of the BGS, to study the health problems and provision of care for the infirm elderly and to recommend suitable solutions. In 1947 the BMA committee issued its report, "The Care and Treatment of the Elderly and Infirm." The report summarized the prevailing widespread neglect of elderly patients in former Poor Law institutions, again noted the threat the inevitable growth of this problem posed for the future hospital resources of the country, and recommended as a solution the establishment for the elderly of coordinated medical services based in general hospitals within health service administrative regions. This forward-looking model service, premised upon comprehensive assessment and rehabilitation and linkages with other sectors of medical and community services, is depicted in the organizational diagram shown in figure 3-1.

The Royal College of Physicians (London) issued a "Report on Provision for the Aged and Infirm," which again identified the problem but did not envision the need to develop special geriatrics units. In at least one documented instance, a leading figure in academic internal medicine, Dr. A. P. Thompson of the University of Birmingham, undertook his own survey of patients in chronic hospitals. He concluded that prevention of the irreversible disability he witnessed lay with incorporating care of the aged, chronically ill patients into the mainstream of general hospital medicine, where they would receive the benefits of modern diagnostic and therapeutic developments. He did not, however, address the need for multidisciplinary services and specifically denied the need for geriatrics specialists (Thompson 1949).

Regional hospital boards were established to manage and develop hospital resources to meet the comprehensive medical needs of their communities in the spirit of the NHS Act. In the absence of any prescribed policy or system for addressing the particular problems of the large numbers of hospitalized elderly they inherited, these authorities allocated resources in varying ways to care of the elderly. The results of this process were assessed in a survey of services for the chronically ill and elderly conducted by the Ministry of Health in 1954–55. A variety of successful and unsuccessful operating conditions were observed among the emerging hospital-based geriatric services. Relatively high turnover in bed use and small or nonexis-

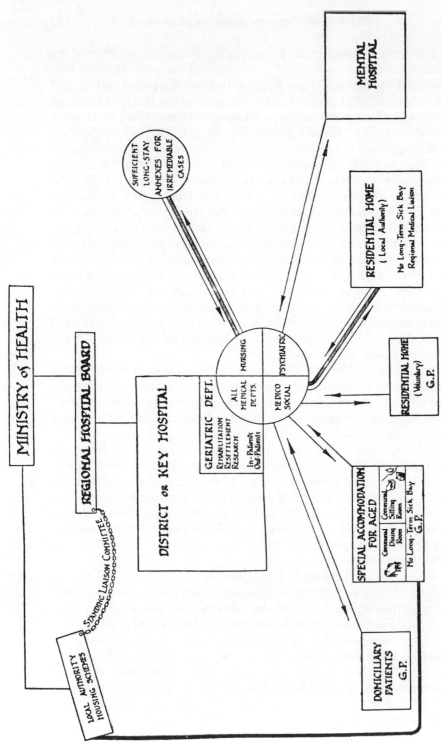

Figure 3-1 The British Medical Association's model of services for the elderly.
Source: British Medical Association. 1947. *The Care and Treatment of the Elderly and Infirm.*
London: British Medical Association. Reprinted with permission.

tent waiting lists of elderly persons referred for chronic hospital care were noted in a few settings that had developed active geriatrics units in line with the BMA model. Factors appearing to contribute to the success of such units included increasing the number of direct referrals from general practitioners, in place of the traditional practice of receiving most patients on transfer from acute wards when they often had little potential for successful rehabilitation; introducing the practice of domiciliary visits by hospital consultants to manage some referrals outside of hospitals; staffing geriatrics wards with medical house officers and remedial therapists to assure prompt assessment and initiation of both acute and rehabilitative care; and appointing full-time geriatrics consultants or equivalent doctors to manage the service. Poor facilities, lack of junior medical staff and rehabilitation therapists, and the tendency to appoint general physicians with mixed commitments to both acute general medicine and geriatrics wards were seen as factors that tended to retard effective development of services (Boucher 1957).

A number of important adjuncts to the active, rehabilitation-oriented aspects of geriatric inpatient services also developed over the years. These include the practice of paying domiciliary visits for initial assessment of patients referred from the community, pioneered by Brook (1948) and Exton-Smith (1952); the development of geriatric day hospitals to assist in transition from inpatient status back to home in the community, originated by the geriatric medicine unit in Oxford (Cosin 1955); the use of some inpatient beds for intermittent respite or holiday admissions to relieve family caretakers (DeLargy 1957); the development of combined geriatric-orthopedic services to improve and expedite hospital care of the growing number of elderly women admitted with hip fractures, a strategy begun in Hastings (Devas 1977); and the very important practice of clearly defining the catchment population of elderly persons to be served by a given geriatrics unit, a concept well demonstrated in the 1950s in the city of Glasgow under the leadership of Dr. Ferguson Anderson (Isaacs, Livingston, and Neville 1972).

The 1960s: The District General Hospital

The years from 1960 to the mid-1970s were a period of major growth in public expenditure in Great Britain. In this era, the Department of Health and Social Security (DHSS) and its Scottish counterpart, the Scottish Home and Health Department (SHHD), undertook their first comprehensive efforts to review extant hospital services and implement a modern hospital plan (Great Britain, Ministry of Health 1962). Underlying this decision were a variety of observations, typified by the detailed surveys of hospital services in the large Birmingham metropolitan area by McKeown and colleagues (personal communication, Dr. Thomas McKeown, April 1983; Lowe and McKeown 1949; McKeown, Mackintosh, and Lowe 1961). They pointed critically to the fact that the hospitals in which patients resided were more a function of outdated, historic precedent than of the type of medical services the patient required. As a case in point, age was noted to be the prime determinant of whether a person requiring full hospital facilities was likely to be located in a general or special hospital (formerly voluntary) or in a hospital for the chronically ill (formerly poorhouse infirmary). This phenomenon is graphically illustrated in figure 3-2, from the Birmingham surveys.

The most significant outcome of the hospital planning movement was the concept of the district general hospital (DGH), an institution that would provide a full range of hospital facilities and specialty services to all persons within an area of 100,000–150,000 persons.

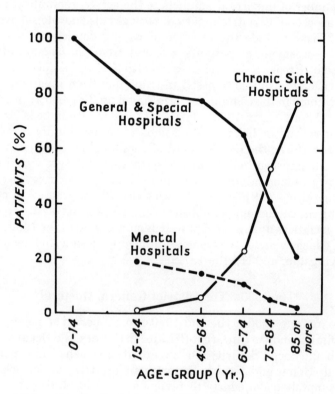

Figure 3-2 Location of patients needing full hospital facilities, by age.
Source: McKeown, T.; Mackintosh, J. M.; and Lowe, C. R. 1961. Influence of age on type of hospital to which patients are admitted. *Lancet* 1:818–20. Reprinted with permission.

Specifically, active psychiatric and geriatric services were to be in-cluded within the DGH, alongside acute medicine and surgery, while long-stay patients might best be cared for in smaller peripheral hos-pitals (Bonham-Carter 1969).

During this period, health service administrators, impressed with the accomplishments of the pioneer geriatrics services of the 1940s and 1950s, actively encouraged the creation of geriatric consultant posts. The composition of services to be under the jurisdiction of these consultants was outlined in a memo entitled "Hospital Geriatric Ser-vices," sent from the Ministry of Health to the Regional Hospital Boards, Boards of Governors of Teaching Hospitals, and Hospital Management Committees in 1971. The memo identified the several levels of care required by infirm elderly patients—acute assessment, rehabilitation, long-term care, intermittent respite care —and recommended that at least 50 percent of geriatric beds be situated in district general hospitals. It also strongly endorsed the establishment of day hospitals as a component of geriatrics services to provide rehabilitation services for elderly patients not requiring hospitalization and for posthospital rehabilitation of inpatients fol-lowing discharge (DHSS 1971).

Concurrent with these national policy developments, professional societies gave their own voice to the movement to improve health services for the elderly. The Royal College of Physicians (RCP) of Edinburgh sponsored two special reports on *Care of the Elderly in Scotland*. The first, in 1963, was charged "to consider the arrange-ments and facilities for the care of the elderly in Scotland and to make recommendations" (p. 9). The report gave strong support to the placement of geriatric assessment and rehabilitation beds in general hospital as "acute" services and to the establishment of consultant as well as junior level hospital posts in geriatric medicine (RCP Edin-burgh 1963). The second report was a follow-up assessment of prog-ress during the decade. The report noted a significant increase in general hospital beds in some but not all regions of Scotland, plus a major increase in full-time geriatrics consultants (from eighteen to thirty-six) and junior level hospital posts (RCP Edinburgh 1972). The Royal College of Physicians of London established a Committee on Geriatric Medicine in 1967, which issued its first report and recom-mendations on developing geriatrics services in England and Wales in 1972. While generally supportive of NHS policy directions, this effort was not as strong as that in Scotland in part because the Royal College, dominated by physicians in internal medicine, was reluctant to endorse the concept of an independent specialty of geriatrics.

In the wake of governmental and professional efforts in the 1960s, the ensuing years have become the era of "modern geriatric medi-

28 Adding Life to Years

cine" in Great Britain. The commitment to this component of health
services is demonstrated by the existence of hospital-based geriatrics
units in virtually all of the several hundred health districts in the
country. The majority of units include admitting beds in general
hospitals, and virtually all include a strong rehabilitation component. The number of geriatric consultant posts approximates five
hundred, and there has been a steady growth in the number of hospital-based training posts allocated to geriatrics (Green 1975;
Brocklehurst and Andrews 1985; Brocklehurst 1984).

The British Geriatrics Society (BGS) has promulgated a number of
recommended norms for district geriatrics services (see Appendix B)
and in collaboration with the Royal College of Nursing (RCN) developed detailed recommendations for equipping and managing hospital geriatrics units (BGS/RCN 1975). These have been widely distributed to NHS regional and local administrators. In 1965 the first
professorship in geriatric medicine was established at the University
of Glasgow, and there are now twelve medical schools with professorial departments. All but two of the medical schools in the country have required that curriculum time be devoted to geriatrics
(Smith and Williams 1983).

Paralleling the growth in the hospital-based and academic aspects
of geriatric medicine has been an emphasis on development of primary medical care, nursing, social work, and remedial therapy services
related to the care of the elderly in the community.* These services
play essential roles complementary to the hospital-based geriatrics
units; they both help patients avoid unnecessary hospital admission
and expedite discharge of patients whose primary needs may be met
in their homes.

To monitor the effectiveness with which geriatrics resources have
been deployed, Hospital Advisory Services for the NHS and the
SHHD have reviewed developments district by district since the late
1960s. Their reports, echoing observations of the 1954–55 survey
cited earlier, have identified the attributes of above-average geriatrics units as summarized in Appendix C. They have also identified
important gaps in services, among the most critical being the con-

*This emphasis is epitomized in "Priorities for Health and Personal Social Services
in England," a health policy consultative document published by the Department of
Health and Social Services in 1976 which contains the leading statement: "The main
objective of services for elderly people is to help them remain in the community for as
long as possible" (p. 38). This document represents a response to the 1974 administrative reorganization of the National Health Service, a major intent of which was to
strengthen coordination between institutional and community services. A British
Medical Association working party report, "Care of the Elderly," also published in
1976, contains many detailed recommendations for strengthening the mix of medical,
nursing, and social services for supporting elderly persons living in their own homes.

tinued location of some district services in outdated facilities and the related difficulty in attracting well-trained medical, nursing, and remedial therapy staff (unpublished periodic reports of the Hospital Advisory Services).

Acute Geriatrics Services

As the demands of an aging population upon acute hospitals intensified in the later 1970s, the role of geriatrics services has increasingly shifted toward more active involvement in acute care. This phenomenon has been acknowledged and encouraged in a series of government consultative documents. It is well summarized in the following excerpt from *Growing Older,* a white paper submitted to Parliament in 1981 by the secretary of state:

> Increasingly, an active approach is being adopted to the treatment and rehabilitation of elderly patients in hospital, which reflects both the best modern practice and the desire of most to return home as soon as possible. The success of modern methods of treatment depends greatly on whether elderly patients are admitted in the first instance to a general hospital where full facilities for diagnosis, treatment and rehabilitation are readily available. Effective management is likely to be best achieved where a department of geriatric medicine is situated in the same building as the other acute specialties. In these circumstances, the consultant physician in geriatric medicine can admit directly any elderly patient who is more likely to respond to treatment and care by his own specially trained, multi-disciplinary team. He can make advice and guidance readily available to other departments, who in turn are able to advise him on problems on which they have particular expertise. The presence of his team in the general hospital also provides a focus for the dissemination to hospital staff (and others in the community) of knowledge and understanding of the special problems associated with the care of elderly people. Within available resources, faster progress needs to be made in the development of units for acute geriatric medicine alongside general acute departments. (P. 51)

Several different operational models for increasing involvement in acute hospital care of the elderly have emerged through the efforts of progressive elements within the geriatric medicine movement. These may be characterized as follows (Barker 1986b):

1. *Selective referral.* A self-contained geriatrics unit that has evolved a policy of encouraging general practitioners and acute hospital colleagues to refer selected patients for consultation at the time of onset of acute problems, rather than waiting until the patients reach a stage of immobility, incontinence, and so forth and are in

need of prolonged rehabilitation. This strategy, which requires good general hospital facilities and an enthusiastic staff, has been reported to increase bed turnover rates, eliminate waiting lists for patients to be seen, and reduce bed blocking in acute units. Examples have been described from several settings (Hodkinson and Jeffries 1972; McAlpine 1979; ch. 4).

2. *Age-related service.* A self-contained geriatrics unit that assumes responsibility for general medical care of virtually all patients over a specified age (e.g., 70 or 75) who are referred to hospital. This model, analagous to pediatrics, assures that all patients who may benefit from the special expertise and services of geriatric medicine will receive them from the outset of hospital referral, along with appropriate acute medical care. High bed turnover rates and elimination of waiting lists are again achieved when this strategy is successfully applied, as described from several settings (O'Brien, Joshi, and Warren 1973; Bagnall et al. 1977).

3. *Integrated service.* A unit that incorporates geriatrics services within the general medicine service of a district general hospital, thereby eliminating the need for two separate administrative structures. Such units are staffed by a team of general medicine consultants, some of whom have special training in care of the elderly, others of whom have special training in other medical subspecialty areas (e.g., cardiology, endocrinology, etc.), or in some instances by physicians with combined training in both geriatrics and an organ system specialty. All of the consultants accept varying degrees of responsibility for elderly as well as nonelderly medical patients referred to hospital; those trained in the care of the elderly take responsibility for most patients requiring rehabilitation and related geriatric expertise. This approach, which is believed to attain optimal use of the limited acute resources of district general hospitals, was pioneered at Oxford and has been developed in other settings, several of which have recently been described (Evans 1983; Evans and Graham 1984).

The evolution of these several active or acute models is still very much in progress, involving a growing but undetermined number of geriatrics units in the country. The selection of one model over another is contingent on local circumstances. For instance, in England, which has traditionally had greater difficulty recruiting candidates to fill geriatric consultant posts than Scotland, regional hospital authorities have been encouraged to evolve integrated services staffed by general physicians with a special responsibility (but not full-time assignment to) geriatrics (DHSS 1979). This concept, first espoused by the RCP London Working Party on Medical Care of the Elderly (1977), has been endorsed in a recent major DHSS consultative document entitled "The Respective Roles of the General Acute and Geriatric Sectors in Care of the Elderly Hospital Patient" (1981b). Scotland, by contrast, in confronting an increasing problem with bed blocking in acute medical services, has been more inclined to seek ways to enhance the involvement of its strong existing geriatrics departments with acute patient care. A variety of such strategies were considered in a symposium sponsored by the RCP Edinburgh in 1980 (RCP Edinburgh 1981).

Comment

Modern geriatric medicine in Great Britain has evolved from its mid–twentieth-century origins in former Poor Law institutions to its current base in the general hospital sector. Hospital-based geriatrics services, organized according to one of several distinctive models for admitting elderly patients and staffed by multidisciplinary teams, including medical specialists, exist in virtually all health districts. While emphasizing early active intervention in treating disease and disability of old age in hospital, geriatrics services have also developed innovative approaches to avoiding hospital admission and expediting discharge from hospital to the community. Furthermore, in keeping with the original work of Marjory Warren, the geriatric medicine movement continues to address institutional health care needs of growing numbers of dependent elderly persons requiring long-term care. Specifically, geriatrics departments have, through mutual agreements with local social service departments, undertaken to provide medical assessment and rehabilitation services to those elderly persons who, for primarily social reasons, are referred to long-stay residential facilities which are outside of the mainstream of medical care. A joint statement prepared in the early 1980s by the British Geriatrics Society and the British Association of Directors of Social Services, who are responsible for these facilities, summarizes this important initiative (see Appendix D). Similarly in response to recent government initiatives to encourage development of private nursing homes (1985) as a means of relieving the growing demands of disabled elderly persons on public long-term care facilities, the British Geriatrics Society has worked actively to establish standards of appropriate medical care for elderly persons in these non–Health Service settings (personal communication, Robert Kandt, British Geriatrics Society, April 1986).

While development of organized geriatrics services has been facilitated by the existence of the British National Health Service and fostered by health policies directed to the needs of the elderly, nonetheless the initiatives of individual leaders and geriatrics units have also played a critical role in developing the field. For purposes of observing the best results of this developmental process, a number of carefully selected sites were visited in compiling the profile of the practice of geriatric medicine found in the following three chapters.

CHAPTER 4

A Model Geriatric Medicine Unit in Edinburgh

Setting

Edinburgh is the principal population center of the Lothian area (total population 748,000), one of fifteen administrative regions of the Scottish Home and Health Department. Geriatrics services in the region are provided by three major units, each of which is based in a hospital in Edinburgh, and two small, rural units in east and west Lothian affiliated with the Edinburgh units. Each unit serves the elderly population of a geographically defined catchment area (see fig. 4-1).

The three Edinburgh units are based at the City Hospital (population of catchment area approximately 19,000 aged 65+), the Longmore Hospital (population of catchment area approximately 26,000 aged 65+), and the Royal Victoria Hospital (population of catchment area approximately 36,000 aged 65+). The Professorial Unit of the University of Edinburgh at the City Hospital served as the primary site for observing and assembling the information that follows. This unit, having major teaching and research commitments in addition to providing direct services, has a smaller catchment population than the other two.

Structure and Staffing

The essential resources of the unit include approximately 240 hospital beds, a small hospital outpatient clinic, and a day hospital with a daily capacity of 30. Forty of the hospital beds are used for acute assessment and rehabilitation. These 40 beds are based at the City Hospital, a former municipal communicable disease hospital that has been modernized to serve as a general hospital, including university departments of respiratory medicine, infectious diseases, ear, nose, and throat, as well as geriatrics. The remaining geriatrics beds are used for long-stay care of patients who are unable to materially benefit from rehabilitation but require continuing nursing care and

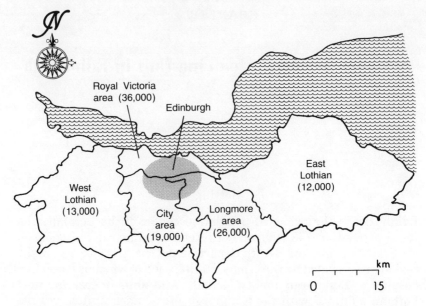

Figure 4-1 Geriatrics unit catchment areas, Lothian Health Board, Scotland.
Adapted from figure furnished by Dr. James Williamson.

medical supervision. These beds are distributed among five hospital sites, one of which is a new 90-bed unit; the other beds are located in older hospitals, several of which have outlived their original purpose (e.g., a former tuberculosis sanatorium).

Jurisdiction over the beds and the general operational policies of the unit is vested in the professor of geriatric medicine and two senior colleagues, all of whom hold National Health Service posts of (honorary) consultants in geriatric medicine along with their academic appointments. (This pattern is common in academic clinical departments in Great Britain, most of which have designated service responsibilities.) Other medical staff members include two senior registrars (comparable to specialty fellows in the United States), who divide their time between teaching, research, and service roles preparatory to seeking career posts as consultants; two registrars (comparable to senior residents in the United States), who primarily supervise and participate actively in day-to-day inpatient care; and three senior house officers (comparable to junior residents in the United States), who as part of their basic training for general medicine or general practice choose rotations on the geriatric inpatient service.

All hospital wards as well as the day hospital are staffed by state-registered nurses (registered nurse equivalent) and state-enrolled nurses (licensed practical nurse equivalent) and are under the general charge of a senior nursing sister. Community nursing services, which are not officially attached to the geriatrics unit but maintain active liaison, particularly in discharge planning, include both district nurses (equivalent to community health visiting nurses), who perform a wide variety of practical nursing functions in patients' homes, and health visitors, who provide assessment and counseling services focused on psychosocial needs of patients living in the community. Most community nurses are attached to specified general practices located within the City Hospital catchment area, hence facilitating coordinated medical and nursing care in the community, as discussed in detail in chapter 7. The assessment and rehabilitation wards and day hospital are staffed by two full-time social workers, several full-time physiotherapists and occupational therapists, a full-time dietician, and a part-time speech therapist. These individuals have decided on a career in geriatrics in their discipline or are spending time in this specialty as part of their training. While all of these health professionals are hired by their respective professional administrative offices of the Lothian Health Board or Social Work Department, their placement and de facto membership in the City Hospital geriatric unit has been successfully negotiated over time. The result is a well-balanced multidisciplinary team to run the unit.

Operational Aspects

Operations of the unit may be divided between the several patient care processes under direct jurisdiction of the unit (referrals, admission, assessment and rehabilitation, discharge, continuing care) and the various consulting activities involving related medical, surgical, and social services. It is the policy of the unit to receive referrals of patients over age 65 who experience acute or progressive changes in health status that are likely to require multidisciplinary assessment and rehabilitation in addition to acute medical care. (These referrals would not generally include life-threatening emergencies such as a heart attack with shock or discrete illnesses such as a bleeding ulcer in an otherwise healthy elderly person; these persons are more appropriately referred to general medicine.) The general policy also encourages referral of families experiencing difficulty with an unhealthy older member. The unit receives some twelve hundred to fifteen hundred direct referrals a year, most of which come from general practitioners whose patients are among the nineteen thousand elderly who reside within the City Hospital geriatric unit catchment area. This translates into a ratio of approximately 4–6 referrals per 100 persons over age 65 in the catchment area per year. A home visit is made on each new referral, usually on the day received. This visit allows the consultant to make a rapid disposition, either to admit the person as an acute patient or to make some alternative arrangement such as referral to day hospital for assessment and rehabilitation.

Once admitted to either hospital or day hospital, patients undergo full medical, functional, and mental status assessment, as indicated for their presenting problem(s), and an appropriate course of medical care; concurrently they are screened by the nursing staff, the social worker, and the physical and occupational therapists to determine which of these respective services are needed. All members of this multidisciplinary team are oriented to achieve the fullest possible restoration of the patient's capacity to function independently and to return to home. The concerns, expectations, and demands of the patient's family and other care givers are addressed as a central part of the process. This rehabilitation orientation may be illustrated by several specific practices. Nurses routinely encourage almost all patients to get out of bed each day, to dress themselves in their own clothes and to walk to the toilet insofar as they are able (in lieu of becoming bedpan dependent). Physiotherapists conduct mobility exercises on the wards in familiar environs, where nurses and other staff can directly observe and reinforce these aspects of patient rehabilitation. To emphasize socialization, tea and meals are served in a day room, with patients sitting at a properly laid table rather than in bed. Occupational therapists and social workers frequently schedule trial home visits for a patient prior to discharge to assess her ability to function in the home environment and to arrange for modification of that environment if necessary. This practice helps reassure family members that the patient can indeed cope at home.

The linchpin of the unit's activities is a weekly multidisciplinary case conference at which each patient's progress is reviewed and next steps in rehabilitation are decided. When a patient is ready for discharge, the consultant, working with colleagues from the other disciplines and their collective knowledge of resources available in the community, has a spectrum of possible dispositions available, including the following:

1. Discharge home, with a letter to the patient's general practitioner regarding diagnosis, medications, and so forth. This disposition is the most common. Concurrently a notification of discharge is relayed by telephone to the district nurse or health visitor attached to the patient's general practice (see ch. 7), and the patient is routinely visited by one of these persons within a few days of discharge. Details of pending patient discharge are often discussed with a liaison community health nurse who participates in the case conferences.

2. Discharge home with planned continuation of rehabilitation and medical treatment in the day hospital. This option allows the geriatrician to discharge patients earlier than might otherwise be the case, with the intent of facilitating transition from hospital to home. Patients typically come to day hospital for a half-day session, including a meal, once or twice per week for about six to eight weeks. Transportation is provided by the health services.

3. Discharge home with arrangement for special services to assist the patient at home. This option may include scheduling meals on wheels, a home help to assist with meals, shopping and other domestic needs, or a domiciliary occupational therapist to provide simple aides and environmental alterations to facilitate bathing, cooking, dressing, and so forth. These services are available through liaison with the area social work office in whose jurisdiction the patient lives.

4. Discharge home with arrangements for periodic readmission to the geriatrics service to provide the patient with proper medical and related supervision while family members take a holiday or respite from meeting their relative's heavy care needs at home.

5. Transfer to one of the geriatrics unit's long-stay beds for continuing nursing and medical supervision. (These facilities are roughly equivalent to skilled nursing facilities in the United States.) Day-to-day medical care in these settings is provided by house officers or general practitioners on a contract basis, under supervision of the geriatric consultants. Most acute medical problems that supervene in these patients are managed within the long-stay area, and referral to acute hospital or back to the geriatric assessment ward is relatively rare (see ch. 6).

6. Discharge to a long-stay residential facility run by the Lothian Social Work Department. Such a facility provides a home for persons who are physically independent but, due to age and/or failing mental status or social circumstances, are unable or unwilling to live at home on their own. (These facilities are roughly equivalent to intermediate care or health-related facilities in the United States).

7. Discharge to a private nursing home or residential accommodation, should the patient have the resources and desire to exercise the option. (There are relatively few private nursing homes in Edinburgh; most are quite small, with a mean capacity of twenty-two patients per home [Primrose and Capewell 1986].)

Several published and unpublished analyses of the aforementioned patient care activities provide graphic insight into selected aspects of the practice of geriatric medicine in Great Britain. An analysis of 209 consecutive home visits in response to general practitioner referrals found that 35 percent of patients were admitted for acute care to the inpatient unit, 31 percent were referred to the day hospital, 11 percent were managed at home by the GP with recommendations, and 23 percent were referred to various other medical specialties or social services (Arcand and Williamson 1981). While these geriatric consultations were sought for a wide range of presenting medical problems, a variety of nonclinical problems were also recorded at the time of the home visits, as enumerated in table 4-1. These observations generally contributed in important ways to decisions regarding immediate and long-term patient management.

Table 4-2, compiled from routinely collected statistics, provides an overall profile of community-dwelling patients referred to the geriatric service and compares those admitted to the acute inpatient hospital unit and the day hospital, respectively. Mean age (80–82 years old), proportion of females (67–70 percent), and proportions with various medical problems were for the most part very similar. The presence of major associated physical disabilities (urinary incontinence, limitation of mobility) and the receipt of home nursing services best distinguished those for whom hospital admission was deemed necessary. This clearly more dependent group of patients

Table 4-1
Nonclinical Problems Observed during 209 Consecutive Visits
to Homes of Elderly Persons

Problems	Percent of Visits
Social	
Neglect of household	9
Poor catering	13
Inadequate heating	9
Interpersonal tension	28
Inadequate social support	35
Approaching or actual family exhaustion	49
Nursing	
Self-neglect	14
Inability to visit essential areas of house	41
Inadequate nursing care	32
Medical	
Poor compliance with a prescribed diet	10
Alcohol abuse	3
Poor compliance with prescribed drug regimen	14
Drugs being taken that were not mentioned by referring general practitioner	23
Prevention and rehabilitation	
Accident hazards	23
Need for special aids	25
Opportunity for patient (or carer) to demonstrate problems within the home, such as difficult stairs, chair or bed too low, etc.	58

Source: Adapted from Arcand and Williamson 1981. Reprinted with permission.

Table 4-2
Selected Characteristics of 473 Consecutive Referrals to Geriatric Inpatient Unit
and Day Hospital

Characteristics	Inpatient Unit	Day Hospital
Number	260	213
Age (mean years)	82	80
Female	67%	70%
Presenting problems		
Musculoskeletal	50%	49%
Cardiovascular	38	36
Urinary incontinence	45	22
Respiratory	28	14
Dementia	29	23
Depression	9	14
Death in 6 months	24%	7%
Mobility		
Unaided	15%	63%
With aid	43	34
Wheelchair/bed bound	42	3
Dwelling		
Home alone	38%	43%
Home with family/other	50	53
Residential home	12	4
Home services		
Home help	39%	47%
District nurse	30	19

Sources: Unpublished study by K. Kieburtz and V. Kieburtz, as well as personal communication, 1985. Reprinted with permission.

experienced a markedly higher mortality rate (personal communication, Kieburtz and Kieburtz 1985).

The dynamics of the department's geriatric day hospital were closely observed during a six-month period. Of 334 persons attending, one-third were referred following a stay in the inpatient geriatrics unit, while most of the remainder were direct referrals from general practitioners. Seventy-four (22 percent) attended only once for assessment and disposition or brief hospital follow-up. Among the 260 who received ongoing day hospital care, 70 percent attended once weekly, 24 percent twice weekly, and 6 percent on various other schedules. Attendance continued over a two- to three-month period for most, with a small percentage receiving long-term continuing care. During their sessions at the day hospital, patients received and participated in various medical and rehabilitative activities; the frequencies are shown in table 4-3 (Martinez, Carpenter, and Williamson 1984).

Table 4-3
Services Provided to 260 Consecutive Patients Referred to Geriatric Day Hospital

Services	Percent
Medical assessment	100
Nursing	
Bowel care	39
Bathing	27
Serial blood pressure	25
Medication supervision	12
Skin ulcer care	7
Catheter care	5
Physical therapy	49
Occupational therapy	70
Chiropody	12
Dietary	20
Social work	
Home visit	15
Residential planning	5

Source: Adapted from Martinez, Carpenter, and Williamson 1984. Reprinted with permission.

Consultative Activities

Consultative liaison with related medical and social services constitutes an important and expanding role whereby the geriatrics unit has amplified the impact of its expertise in the community. From its inception in 1976 as an academic department with service responsibilities, it was agreed that the City Hospital geriatrics unit, along with the other two Edinburgh geriatrics units, would provide consultative services to the large general medicine service in the Royal Infirmary of Edinburgh, the university's major teaching hospital (personal communication, Dr. Ian Campbell, former chief medical officer, Lothian Health Board, February 1983). Accordingly, a system was implemented whereby a geriatric consultant visits each of four medical wards twice a week to consult on any newly admitted elderly patients who are likely to require rehabilitation or continuing care or whose return to home in the community may be problematical. This arrangement brings geriatrics skills, precepts, and practices to the acute sector. A multidisciplinary discussion of these patients is conducted on site, and recommendations are provided for the attending staff. Patients are reevaluated each week until discharge, but they are rarely transferred to the geriatrics unit.

In the first full year of operation, this consult service provided by the City Hospital unit reviewed 255 men and 314 women, representing, respectively, 61 percent and 70 percent of all elderly patients admitted to the general medicine wards to which they were attached. Average lengths of stay were significantly reduced in comparison with the prior year's experience, as discussed in detail in chapter 6 (Burley et al. 1979). (In spite of these efforts, which have had a documented impact in decreasing patient length of stay, the general medical services continue to have beds "blocked" by elderly patients. The management team of the Royal Infirmary has therefore recommended the opening of a geriatrics service to admit acutely ill elderly persons directly from the emergency room. This strategy, similar to one successfully implemented elsewhere in Great Britain [see ch. 6], would provide intensive application of geriatric practices from the outset of hospitalization, with the intention of reducing the number of patients who reach the "bed-blocking" state on general medicine units.)

In 1978 an analogous consultation liaison was established between the geriatric medicine department and the acute orthopedic surgery unit at the Royal Infirmary. In this case the geriatric consultant visits elderly orthopedic patients, primarily women with hip fractures, shortly after admission and arranges by mutual agreement with the orthopedic unit to take joint responsibility for the postoperative care of those patients with special geriatric rehabilitation needs. For this phase of care the patient is transferred to a special Geriatric-Orthopedic Rehabilitation Unit (GORU) located at the nearby Princess Margaret Rose Orthopedic Hospital. In this setting, a consultant geriatrician has overall responsibility for medical care and runs a weekly multidisciplinary case conference where rehabilitation and discharge plans are discussed (Burley 1983). Because this activity has expedited acute and rehabilitative hospital care of elderly orthopedic patients, a new geriatric consultant post was recently approved by the Lothian Health Board to expand this service to cover a larger proportion of such patients (personal communication, Dr. Joseph McMillan, Hospital Planning, Lothian Health Board, May 1983).

Geriatric psychiatry services are provided to geographically defined catchment areas in Edinburgh in a fashion roughly similar to the geriatric medicine units. The service in the City Hospital catchment area is based at the Royal Edinburgh Hospital, a large psychiatric facility that houses the university Department of Psychiatry. The service is staffed by psychiatrists, with primary responsibility for the mentally ill elderly, and a number of psychiatric nurses, social workers, and remedial therapists. Facilities include two new day hospitals, a modern inpatient assessment and rehabilitation unit, and long-stay beds. Like the geriatric medicine unit, the psychogeriatrics unit receives referrals primarily from general practitioners. While these elderly patients commonly have chronic physical health problems, they are referred to psychiatry when their

2

primary active problem is in the mental health domain. Tables 4-4
and 4-5 show reasons for referral and diagnostic classification among
one hundred consecutive referrals to the Royal Edinburgh Hospital
psychogeriatrics unit (Boyd, Woodside, and Zealley 1979). At the
present time this service and the geriatric medicine unit consult with
each other on an ad hoc basis regarding the management of individual patients.

Relationships with general practitioners, of whom there are about
ninety who regularly refer patients to the City Hospital geriatrics
unit, have been developed primarily through consultations on individual patients. The unit also hosts an annual gathering for GPs to
review the past year's experience, discuss new components of the
service that may have been developed, and entertain questions and
suggestions.

Extensive liaison exists between the geriatrics unit and the
Lothian Department of Social Work, particularly through the contribution of the social workers to the discharge planning process discussed earlier. Social services critical to effective functioning of the
geriatric medicine unit include long-stay residential facilities, to
which a small number of medically stable geriatric inpatients are
discharged each year, and community-based social work offices that
deploy home helps, meals on wheels, domiciliary occupational therapists, and general purpose caseworkers to patients' homes as needed.
One or more of these services is provided as part of the initial disposition on 25 percent or more of all patients seen by the geriatrics unit
on referral from the community. The geriatricians in turn routinely

Table 4-4

Reasons for Consultation on 100 Consecutive Patients Referred to
Psychogeriatrics Service

Reasons	Percent
Aggressive/violent/unmanageable	25
Confusion	15
Confused and delusional	14
Demented	10
Loss of memory	9
Wandering out of house	9
Depression	8
Doubly incontinent (relative/wife cannot cope)	6
Not eating/drinking/staying in bed	4
Suicidal attempts/threats	3
Alcoholism/disturbed behavior	2
Miscellaneous	4
No reason recorded	3

Source: Adapted from Boyd, Woodside, and Zeally 1979. Reprinted with permission.
Note: A few patients appear in more than one category.

Table 4-5
Initial Diagnostic Classification of 100 Consecutive Patients Referred to
Psychogeriatrics Service

Diagnostic Classification	Percent
Dementias	59
Affective disorder	14
Paranoid reactions	7
Acute confusional states	3
Alcoholism	2
No psychiatric diagnosis made	15
TOTAL	100

Source: Adapted from Boyd, Woodside, and Zeally 1979. Reprinted with permission.

provide preadmission assessment of patients in their catchment area who are referred directly to the Social Work Department by their general practitioner for admission to a long-term residential accommodation. This assessment is intended to detect and address any remedial medical or physical disorders prior to placement. The unit performs between 100 to 150 such assessments each year. A retrospective analysis of approximately 700 of these assessments over a number of years revealed that about 10 percent were referred for medical treatment in the geriatrics unit or elsewhere, while the rest were in stable medical status (Rafferty, Smith, and Williamson 1987).

Education and Research

In its academic capacity, the Department of Geriatric Medicine at the University of Edinburgh is actively engaged in both teaching and research. Teaching includes undergraduate and postgraduate medical education as well as ad hoc teaching arrangements with nursing and rehabilitation therapy students and various community groups. Undergraduate medical education consists of a four-week required clinical course that includes one week of seminars and field trips to introduce major geriatric health problems and components of geriatrics services and three weeks of clinical clerkship attached to an approved geriatrics unit in Edinburgh or elsewhere in the south of Scotland. Graduate education consists of several years of training in general hospital medicine, including successfully writing the exam for Membership in the Royal College of Physicians (analogous to board certification in internal medicine in the United States), and two or more years of training as registrar and senior registrar in geriatric medicine (see ch. 8 for further discussion of medical education and graduate training in geriatric medicine).

The department has been actively involved in two particularly innovative undertakings in postgraduate or continuing medical education. First is the establishment in 1983 of a School of Primary Health Care in the Elderly to provide short courses and study days for GPs, nurses, and other community-based health professionals. The focus is upon practical diagnostic and multidisciplinary management strategies in caring for the elderly in the community. Table 4-6 lists a number of topic areas covered in these courses. A book on this experience has recently been published (Williamson et al. 1986).

Second is the department's leadership in developing and coordinating a two-week course entitled The Aging of Populations: Clinical Care of the Elderly, largely intended for physicians from other countries with an interest in geriatrics. Sponsored by the British Council, a nonprofit organization for the dissemination of information on British culture, the course is designed to present the state of the art of geriatric medicine and geriatric health services, as evolved in Great Britain. The composition of the course has been described and highly lauded by former participants (Schler, Erickson, and Stickler 1985).

The faculty have undertaken a wide range of research projects in the areas of health service delivery, medical education, clinical geriatrics, and epidemiology. Most of the studies have been generated from observations and inquiries arising directly out of day-to-day service and teaching activities, hence the findings have often been directly applicable to improving geriatrics services in Edinburgh and elsewhere.

An early and sustained interest in "preventive geriatrics" has resulted in a series of observational and intervention studies, several of which are discussed in chapter 7. Other descriptive and evaluative

Table 4-6
Sample Course of Instruction in Primary Health Care for the Elderly,
Department of Geriatric Medicine, University Of Edinburgh

Day	Curriculum Topics	Day	Curriculum Topics
Day 1	The elderly in the community and institutions	Day 3	Psychiatric problems
	Demography		Dementias
	Elderly living alone		Depression, paranoia
	Elderly in institutions		Psychogeriatric services
Day 2	Presenting problems in old age	Day 4	Services for the elderly
	Atypical presentation of disease		Social services
	Clinical assessment		Acute hospital
	Pharmacology		Augmented home care

Source: Personal communication, Dr. James Williamson, April 1985.
Note: All sessions include lecture and case presentations.

health service delivery studies of day hospital and liaison activities with medicine and orthopedic surgery are discussed earlier in this chapter and in chapter 6. In the clinical realm, the department has been particularly interested in drug use and adverse drug reactions among the elderly (Williamson and Chopin 1980; Stephen and Williamson 1984). Members of the department have coauthored two recent national studies dealing with education and training, one a survey of medical school curriculum in geriatrics in Great Britain (Smith and Williams 1983), the other a survey of career development patterns among recently appointed consultants in geriatric medicine (Barker and Williamson 1986). These are discussed in detail in chapter 8. Finally, epidemiologic study of a cohort of some five hundred community-dwelling elderly persons, who were systematically observed for a number of years beginning in 1966, has resulted in a series of forty-six published papers on incidence, prevalence, and clinical patterns of common medical, physical, and mental health problems of aging. These studies, along with a detailed description of the research methodology, have been published in a single volume entitled *Clinical Effects of Aging: A Longitudinal Study* (Milne 1985).

Comment

The structure, staffing, and operation of the geriatric medicine unit based at the City Hospital in Edinburgh illustrate the organized continuum of services that comprise modern geriatrics units in Great Britain. While based in a general hospital with responsibility for an acute admitting service as well as a day hospital and long-stay beds, the unit also works through active liaisons with other hospital services and community-based general practitioners, nursing, and social services. Virtually all clinical activities include a multidisciplinary, rehabilitative orientation along with attention to the strictly biomedical aspects of health and disease. In its additional role as the locus of the University of Edinburgh Department of Geriatric Medicine, the unit provides a full array of undergraduate and postgraduate education and has sponsored many published clinical, epidemiological, and health services studies, which have contributed importantly to the academic identity of the field of geriatric medicine.

CHAPTER 5

Elements of the Geriatrics Model
in Twenty Different Settings

Sites Visited

Visits to selected geriatric medicine units throughout Great Britain were undertaken to determine how the basic elements of modern geriatrics services, as described in the literature and observed in Edinburgh, have been implemented in various settings. While looking for commonalities, local variations on the theme were fully anticipated and sought. Information in this chapter and in chapter 6 was initially compiled from semistructured interviews with the hosts and others at each site, as outlined in Appendix E. These interviews were supplemented by copious reading materials, including many unpublished internal documents furnished during or following the visits. A preliminary draft of information contained in these chapters was then reviewed by each of the hosts for accuracy and completeness. This chapter discusses the structural and operational features observed among the units.

Figure 5-1 shows the locations of the sites visited: 2 in Wales, 4 in Scotland (including the Edinburgh unit), 5 in greater London, and 9 elsewhere in England. Table 5-1 lists selected features of each unit, beginning with official department title, names of health districts served, size of the population 65 years of age or above, and classification according to admission policy. The majority of the 20 units visited serve the elderly populace of a single geographically defined health district. This pattern applies among both teaching units in large metropolitan areas (London, Glasgow, Edinburgh) and nonteaching units in relatively discrete communities such as Great Yarmouth, Oldham, and Wrexham. In some instances (Nottingham, Cardiff, Hull, and Oxford) the geriatrics unit serves multiple health districts. District maps and census data, such as shown in figure 4-1, were regularly available for defining geographic and demographic characteristics of the catchment area served by each unit.

46

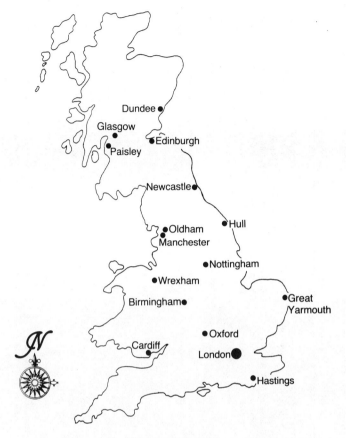

Figure 5-1 Locations of geriatrics units visited.

Staffing and Resources

Most units were staffed by two to four consultants in geriatric medicine; however the number ranged as high as five and seven in two
large units based in university departments at Cardiff and Nottingham. The ratio of consultants to unit of population over age 65
approximated 1:10,000–15,000 in most instances. Some of the uni-
versity-based departments had a lower ratio because up to 50 percent
of the consultants' time was allocated for teaching and research.
Most units had at least one senior registrar as well as one or more
registrars (roughly comparable with subspecialty fellows and senior
residents, respectively, in the United States) plus a number of house
officers. House officers generally rotated through the geriatrics department as part of their general medicine training or as part of the
hospital component of training for general practice. University de-

Table 5-1
Selected Descriptors of Twenty Geriatrics Units Visited during 1983

Descriptors	Birmingham	Cardiff	Charing Cross (London)	Dundee	Edinburgh	Glasgow	Hammersmith (London)	Hastings	Hull	Manchester
Setting										
Department and health district	Dept. Geriatric Medicine South Birmingham Health District	Dept. Clinical Gerontology South Glamorgan Health Authority	Dept. Geriatric Medicine Hammersmith and Fulham Health Authority	Dept. Geriatric Medicine Dundee Health District	Dept. Geriatric Medicine Southwest Lothian Health Board	Dept. Geriatric Medicine Glasgow North Division	Geriatric Med. Unit Hammersmith Health District	Dept. Medicine for the Elderly Hastings Health Authority	Dept. Medicine for the Elderly Hull Health Authority	Dept. Geriatric Medicine Manchester Health Authority, S. District
Population $\geq$ 65	65,000	56,000	17,000	28,000	19,000	30,000	18,000	41,000	68,000	36,000
Admission policy	Selective referral	Age-related	Selective referral	Selective referral	Selective referral	Selective referral	Selective referral	Age-related	Age-related	Selective referral
Medical staffing										
Consultants	3.5 (1)	4 (1)	2	3	3 (3)	4	2 (1)	2	4	5 (2)
Sr. registrars	3 (2)	3 (2)	1	2	2 (1)	2	1	1	2	3 (1)
Registrars	—	5	1	2	2	4	1.5	1	2	2
Hse. officers	6	19	1	4	3	6	3	3	12	5
Hospital resources										
Total beds	500 (7.7)	450 (8.0)	126 (7.4)	418 (14.9)	281 (14.8)	452 (15.1)	127 (7.1)	300 (7.3)	430 (6.3)	310 (8.6)
Beds in DGH	100 (1.5)	223 (4.0)	79 (4.6)	24 (0.9)	40 (2.1)	234 (7.8)	56 (3.1)	142 (3.5)	430 (6.3)	66 (1.8)
DH places	150 (2.3)	115 (2.1)	20 (1.2)	30 (1.1)	30 (1.6)	80 (2.7)		36 (0.9)	120 (1.8)	30 (0.8)
Relations with other depts.										
Medicine	Ad hoc consults	Ad hoc consults	Ad hoc consults	Routine rounds	Routine rounds	Routine rounds	Ad hoc consults	Routine rounds	Ad hoc consults	Ad hoc consults
Orthopedics	Routine transfer	Routine rounds	Ad hoc consults	Routine rounds	GORU	Routine rounds	Routine rounds	GORU	Ad hoc consults	GORU
Psychiatry	Joint service	Routine rounds	Ad hoc consults	Ad hoc consults	Ad hoc consults	Routine rounds	Ad hoc consults	Routine rounds	Ad hoc consults	Routine rounds

Table 5-1 (Continued)
Selected Descriptors of Twenty Geriatrics Units Visited during 1983

Descriptors	Newcastle	Nottingham	Oldham	Oxford	Paisley	St. George's (London)	St. Pancras (London)	West Middlesex (London)	Wrexham	Yarmouth
Setting										
Department and health district	Dept. Medicine (Geriatrics) Newcastle Health Authority	Dept. Health Care of the Elderly Nottingham Health Authority	Dept. Geriatric Medicine Oldham Health Authority	Dept. Geriatric Medicine Oxfordshire Health Authority	Dept. Geriatric Medicine Clyde Health Board, Renfrew District	Dept. Geriatric Medicine Wandsworth Health Authority	Dept. Geriatric Medicine S. Camden Health District	Geriatric Service Hounslow and Spelthorne Authority	Dept. Geriatric Medicine Clwyd, S. District	Geriatric Medicine Great Yarmouth-Waveny Health District
Population ≥ 65	53,000	100,000	32,000	70,000	28,000	28,000	26,000	32,000	30,000	25,000
Admission policy	Integrated with medicine	Selective referral	Age-related	Integrated with medicine	Selective referral	Selective referral	Selective referral	Selective referral	Age-related	Integrated with medicine
Medical staffing										
Consultants	5 (2)	7 (1)	3	4	2	5	2 (1)	2	2	5 med/ger
Sr. registrars	4 (1)	5 (1)	1	4	—	3	3 (1)	1	1	5
Registrars	2	3	1	1	—	2	—	2	2	2
Hse. officers	6	10	5	6	5	11	3	4.5	3	4
Hospital resources										
Total beds	375 (7.1)	550 (5.5)	268 (8.4)	365 (5.2)	402 (14.4)	362 (12.9)	99 (3.8)	204 (6.4)	290 (9.7)	250 (10.0)
Beds in DGH	110 (2.0)	240 (2.4)	218 (6.8)	?	118 (4.2)	76 (2.7)	79 (3.0)	143 (4.5)	99 (3.3)	55 med/ger
DH places	80 (1.5)	55 (0.6)	45 (1.4)	45 (0.6)	—	27 (0.9)	35 (1.3)	22 (0.7)	31 (1.0)	25 (1.0)
Relations with other depts.										
Medicine	Joint service	Ad hoc consults	Ad hoc consults	Joint service	Routine transfer	Ad hoc consults	Routine rounds	?	Ad hoc consults	Joint service
Orthopedics	Ad hoc consults	GORU	Ad hoc consults	Ad hoc consults	Routine transfer	Routine rounds	Ad hoc consults	Joint service	Ad hoc consults	?
Psychiatry	Ad hoc consults	Joint service	Ad hoc consults	Ad hoc consults	Ad hoc consults	Joint service	Routine rounds	?	Routine rounds	?

Notes: Numbers in parentheses under "Medical staffing" indicate consultants and senior registrars with primary academic appointments; numbers in parentheses under "Hospital resources" indicate beds or places per 1,000 population ≥ 65 years of age; DGH = district general hospital; DH = day hospital; GORU = geriatric orthopedic rehabilitation unit; ? = information not obtained.

partments tended to have more senior registrars relative to population served because these posts included academic as well as service commitments. The largest number of house officers relative to population served were found in units with age-related or integrated admission policies which by their nature had the highest acute admission rates. All units had an adequate though not necessarily optimal complement of physical, occupational, and speech therapists and social workers.

The absolute number of hospital beds ranged from 120 to over 500; ratios of beds per 1,000 persons over age 65 ranged from 4 to 15, with more favorable ratios prevailing in Scotland. In all instances, the beds were physically located in multiple hospital sites, including various mixes of district general, rehabilitation, and long-stay hospitals. All units had one or more day hospitals, usually attached to or proximal to one of their inpatient services.

The dynamic state of development of geriatrics resources in Great Britain was evident in a number of instances of current or planned growth, some of which are noted here. Plans were in progress or recently completed to open acute admission geriatrics wards in the major teaching hospitals of the following universities: Edinburgh, Dundee, Nottingham, Oxford, and University College, London. Large new or upgraded geriatrics sections in district general hospitals were soon to be opened in Paisley, West Middlesex, and Wrexham. Application to create new geriatric consultant posts were recently approved by health authorities in Edinburgh, Great Yarmouth, and Nottingham, while applications to establish new posts were pending at several other sites.

The many operational aspects of the units may be subsumed under the following four broad areas: admission policy, discharge planning, deployment of hospital and day hospital facilities, and relationships with other general hospital services.

Hospital Admission and Discharge

Admission policy is largely defined by the type of operational model adopted by the unit, as reviewed in chapter 3. However, some interesting variations in the means of implementing these models were noted. The majority of "selective referral" units have actively fostered direct referrals from general practitioners versus the traditional geriatric role of primarily admitting patients on transfer from other hospital services. The rationale is that direct referral enhances the likelihood that high-risk elderly patients will receive early and optimal diagnosis, medical treatment, and initiation of rehabilitation and require a shorter overall length of inpatient stay. Such strategies have been developed through active outreach to GPs and to emergency room admitting staff on the part of geriatricians. These geriatrics units in turn tend to tightly limit the number of transfer patients they will accept from other hospital services. As an alternative, they have attempted to meet the needs of these patients by providing consultation to other hospital services, as described subsequently. (The geriatric unit in Paisley is an exception to this pattern, having developed a strategy of early referral and transfer from other hospital acute admitting services as a major mode for practicing vigorous and effective rehabilitation, while preventing bed blocking [McAlpine 1979].)

The practice of preadmission assessment is employed to varying degrees among these units. The University of Edinburgh unit stands at one extreme, with a consultant geriatrician making a home visit to virtually every newly referred patient, as described in chapter 4. The rationale is that such visits provide important insight into home conditions, which is important for full assessment and care of the problems of an elderly person. At the other extreme are those units that provide no preadmission visits, preferring to make all assessments and dispositions from within their hospital base. Most selective referral units prefer to use the preadmission assessment visit selectively where they feel it is indicated, and in some instances visiting nurses attached to the unit have been specially trained to perform this role (Pathy, Hughes, and White 1972).

"Age-related" units by definition admit virtually all patients above a designated threshold age who are referred to hospital for general medical care. Threshold age varies among the units visited, from age 65 in Oldham to 75 in Hull and 76 in Hastings. The majority of admitted patients tend to have relatively short lengths of stay for acute problems, while a small percentage resemble the mix of patients admitted to selective referral services, most of whom require extended hospital stay for rehabilitation in addition to initial acute care.

"Integrated" units admit all adult medical referrals, regardless of age, much as is the case in a department of medicine in an acute hospital in the United States. Under these circumstances, any patient may initially be under the care of a consultant in general medicine who has a special interest in one of a variety of specialty areas including geriatric medicine. Following the acute phase of care, those elderly patients requiring rehabilitation or long-term care are transferred to wards designed and staffed for these purposes, under the supervision of the consultant with special interest in geriatrics. In the Newcastle experience, which has been well described, approximately 6 percent of elderly hospitalized patients require such postacute geriatric inpatient care (Evans 1983).

Discharge planning is a very active, critical aspect of a dynamic geriatrics service and generally begins within the first few days of a patient's admission. The essential forum for conducting this activity is a formal multidisciplinary review of each patient one or more times a week. This activity occurs in all units, most commonly taking the form of a case conference presided over by the consultant in geriatric medicine. Each patient's progress and potential toward achieving optimal independent functioning is reviewed and appropriate timing and destination for discharge are discussed in light of current assessment of the patient's status by all involved disciplines (medicine, nursing, physiotherapy, occupational therapy, social work, etc.). Potential arrangements available to all units either directly or through liaison with community nursing or social work services include discharge to home with scheduled follow-up at the geriatric day hospital; arrangements for community nursing services and/or home help (domestic) services in cooperation with the patient's general practitioner; scheduled readmission to provide respite relief for family; or application for admission to a long-stay hospital under the geriatrics department or a residential home for the aged run by the social services, churches, or private parties in the community. To assure smooth transition to home, trial patient home visits with an occupational therapist and/or social worker are selectively utilized by most units.

Deployment of Resources

Hospital beds under jurisdication of geriatric consultants were used to meet medical and medically related needs of the elderly for emergency care, assessment and rehabilitation, long-stay or continuing care, and intermittent respite or holiday admission. Emergency admission beds, including intensive care facilities, were effectively confined to the age-related and integrated geriatrics departments. They were staffed and run by registrars, senior house officers, and registered nurses, and their staffing patterns were indistinguishable from those of acute general medical services. Assessment and rehabilitation beds constituted the mainstay of effort of all geriatrics departments. In addition to accommodating a variety of explicit rehabilitation practices, the environment of these wards was imbued with a rehabilitation atmosphere. Patients were almost always fully dressed in their own footwear and clothing, were out of bed and ambulating or congregating for meals in a day room, and were using toilets rather than becoming dependent upon bedpans or indwelling urinary catheters.

Continuing care beds were occupied by patients who, following full assessment and effort at rehabilitation under a geriatrician's supervision, were judged in need of permanent supportive nursing care and unable to return to the community. Day-to-day medical care was usually provided under contract by general practitioners, while geriatric consultants or senior registrars retained overall responsibility for these patients. Most acute medical problems were handled within the long-stay setting, hence referral of these patients for admission to general hospital was reported to be a rare occurrence, for example, when necessary as in the case of a hip fracture. Reality orientation activities were noted in several long-stay facilities. The geriatrics department at St. George's Medical School has studied the beneficial effects of the presence of long-stay patients' personal belongings (Millard and Smith 1981) and is currently investigating the costs and benefits of personalized single-room long-stay accommodations.

The deployment of 5–10 percent of rehabilitation or continuing care beds for respite or holiday admissions was a universal practice among the departments visited. With average stays of two to three weeks for such admissions, the geriatrics unit is able to provide an essential relief to family, hence maintaining in the community patients who might otherwise require permanent institutional care.

The bed complements of the departments were organized in various patterns to provide the several types of care. Most unusual was the undifferentiated arrangement observed in Hull, where acute care, rehabilitation, and long-stay and respite patients were mixed together in 20- to 30-bed wards throughout the department's approximately 430 beds, all of which were located in one of four district hospitals (Bagnall et al. 1977). It is the prevailing philosophy that in such an atmosphere the more disabled patients will benefit from the active assessment-rehabilitation environment. At the other end of the spectrum are those departments in Cardiff, Hastings, South Manchester, and several others, where acute assessment, rehabilitation, and long-stay beds are separated into a system of progressive care in which patients may be transferred from one setting to another as deemed appropriate by the geriatric consultant. The Hastings experience has been reported, including a review of the concept (Irvine 1963). The rehabilitative components were the most distinctive in such systems, consisting of relatively spacious quarters with areas for occupational and physical therapy and often a section designated specifically for stroke patients. A middle ground was occupied by units such as that at City Hospital in Edinburgh which

Table 5-2

Organizational Patterns of Major Service Components among 220 Geriatrics Units
in Great Britain

Pattern	Percent
Combined acute and rehabilitation; separate long term	38
Separate acute, rehabilitation, long term	24
Combined acute, rehabilitation, long term	21
Separate acute; combined rehabilitation and long term	8
Rehabilitation and long term only	2
Other	7

Source: Adapted from Brocklehurst and Andrews 1985. Reprinted with permission.

combined assessment and rehabilitation within their district general hospital wards, while long-stay beds were located elsewhere. As summarized in table 5-2, this variety of organizational patterns is mirrored in the findings of a nationwide survey of all geriatrics departments conducted by Brocklehurst and Andrews (1985).

An essential administrative component in every geriatrics department is the "bed bureau," where the current census of patients and their level-of-care status can be regularly monitored. This information is commonly displayed on a highly visible master bed board which allows the geriatricians to quickly ascertain how many beds are occupied by persons awaiting discharge, on respite status, and so forth, and to in turn estimate number of vacancies for new admissions. The administrative and related operational aspects of modern geriatrics units have been well described by Pathy (1982) in a book entitled *Establishing a Geriatric Service.*

The Day Hospital

The geriatric day hospital was introduced in Oxfordshire in the 1950s as an adjunct to inpatient geriatric services (Cosin 1955) and has become an essentially universal component of geriatrics departments in Britain (Brocklehurst and Tucker 1980). Its overriding raison d'être is to reduce or prevent hospital stays by providing a variety of medical, rehabilitative, and social services that might otherwise require a person to be in hospital. Medical and nursing services observed in various day hospitals included evaluating patients with recurrent falls, titrating drug regimens for patients with unstable Parkinson's disease, providing bladder and bowel care, and managing chronic varicose ulcers. Rehabilitation activities included, in physiotherapy, reinforcement of gait exercises and training in how to right oneself following a fall and, in occupational therapy, assessment and instruction in activities of daily living (e.g., kitchen skills, dressing, etc.). Social and psychological care included sharing in games, exercises, meals, and other forms of social activity with other patients. Continuation of rehabilitation after hospital discharge to assure successful return to community living was the prime role of the day hospital in most of the settings visited, with patients typically attending one to three times per week for six to ten weeks. Exceptions were noted in Oldham, which supplemented its busy age-related inpatient service with relatively heavy use of its day hospital for medical diagnostic and therapeutic services in lieu of hospital admission. By contrast, the age-related service in Hull tended to draw relatively heavily on its day hospital to provide long-term supportive care in the community for patients with major disability who would otherwise require long-stay hospital beds, which were in short supply in that district. Transportation to and from home to the day hospital was usually provided for free by the National Health Service.

A number of critical reviews have considered the staffing, operational standards, and cost-effectiveness aspects of day hospitals. The consensus has been that when used judiciously, the service unquestionably yields good value for money (Irvine 1980; Hildick-Smith 1984).

Relationships of Geriatric Medicine Departments with Other Hospital Services

In meeting the overall need of hospitalized elderly patients for rehabilitation and long-term disposition, geriatric medicine departments have developed various liaison relationships with other hospital-based departments to which disabled elderly patients tend to be admitted (principally general medicine, orthopedic surgery, and psychiatry). These relationships may be divided into three levels of formality as follows:

1. *Ad hoc consultation,* in which case a geriatric consultant or senior registrar sees individual patients on one of the other services only on special written request from another consultant. This is the least structured and probably least effective liaison arrangement in that patients will often only come to geriatric attention relatively late in their acute hospital course, at which time potential for early initiation of rehabilitation and discharge planning may have been lost.

2. *Routinely scheduled consultation,* in which case the geriatric consultant or senior registrar makes rounds in other departments regularly, one or more times a week, to see any newly admitted elderly patients who may require assessment and advice on diagnosis,

rehabilitation, or long-term care arrangements. This procedure allows recommendations for rehabilitative care and discharge planning to be initiated early in the course of acute hospitalization and also provides reasonable assurance that all patients in need of such care will be identified. This strategy has the limitation of not placing these patients directly under the care of a geriatrics unit, with its pervasive, multidisciplinary rehabilitation orientation.

3. *Joint services,* in which case the geriatrics service and one of the other hospital specialties agree to jointly staff wards that admit patients requiring their respective services. Under these circumstances, the benefits of geriatric rehabilitative care may be realized in a setting other than a pure geriatrics unit.

Among the twenty geriatrics departments visited, all had developed active liaison with one or more other hospital specialty departments. The following table shows the distribution of types of liaison relationships that were observed with medicine, orthopedics, and psychiatry.

Service	Ad Hoc Consults	Routine Consults	Joint Services
Medicine	10	6	3
Orthopedics	7	4	6
Psychiatry	9	6	3

All but one of the geriatrics departments maintained some form of liaison with departments of medicine, with three, as discussed earlier, consisting of joint or integrated departments. Routine consultation rounds were a relatively recent occurrence in several settings, following the reported successes of the prototype experience at the University of Edinburgh in the late 1970s (Burley et al. 1979; see ch. 6).

Liaison with orthopedic surgery departments has occurred in response to the large numbers of elderly women hospitalized with hip fractures ("The Old Woman with a Broken Hip" 1982). These patients typically have coexisting medical and rehabilitative needs that may lead to unnecessarily prolonged hospital stays and bed blocking in orthopedic departments. The concept of a combined geriatric-orthopedic rehabilitation unit to expedite hospital care of these patients was conceived by an orthopedic surgeon, M. B. Devas, in Hastings, where he and physician colleagues responsible for the geriatric unit started the first such service over twenty years ago (Devas 1977). This service and a few others currently exist as fully joint enterprises between the two disciplines, while one more commonly finds geriatrics departments providing either ad hoc or routine consultations to orthopedic departments.

Liaison with psychiatry departments was noted in most units visited, largely dependent on whether the relatively young specialty of psychogeriatrics was represented in the health district (Wattis, Wattis, and Arie 1981). Such liaisons are mutually beneficial: geriatricians are not uncommonly faced with a patient whose primary physical problem is accompanied by difficult-to-manage depression or psychosis, while psychogeriatricians encounter significant numbers of patients whose predominantly mental impairments are accompanied by physical problems, such as incontinence or arthritis, in need of medical attention. The most advanced organizational approach to meeting these mutual needs was noted in the Department of Health Care of the Elderly in Nottingham, where geriatrics and psychogeriatrics are administratively combined, hence facilitating frequent cross-consultation in patient care (Arie 1983). Schemes for routinely scheduled consultation were noted at a number of other sites; an excellent example at the University of Manchester has been described in detail (Jolley et al. 1982).

The Evolution of Units

The evolution of the various geriatrics units that were visited reveals certain common patterns characteristic of the initial post-1948 geriatric medicine movement in Great Britain at large, as well as certain individualized developments reflective of the process of decision making at regional and local levels in recent years. These phenomena are briefly reviewed and illustrated.

The origins of the units could usually be traced to the decisive moment when, in 1948, the NHS assumed responsibility for the chronic care hospitals and their burden of elderly, disabled patients. Typically each of the units began in old and crowded infirmary buildings, with large numbers of beds occupied by custodial care patients and a growing list of other candidates waiting for these beds. The original consultants recruited to the units were, with a few notable exceptions discussed in chapter 3, often semiretired surgeons or former military medical officers, few with training in modern hospital medicine. The major accomplishment of the first phase was to open the beds through introducing rehabilitation and to begin to reduce the waiting lists by visiting and assessing the patients in their homes.

By the 1960s and early 1970s, when the importance of locating geriatrics services in general hospitals had been clearly articulated as an integral part of national hospital planning and policy, geriatrics departments responded in varying ways. Some changed relatively little, carrying on what may be called traditional "slow stream" geriatrics as described above; others, such as the twenty sites selected for this study, underwent active, sometimes dramatic evolution toward a "fast stream" modern form of hospital-based geriatric practice, assuming one of the three operational models described in chapter 3. These developments have been guided and abetted, but not prescribed, by government health policy* and by norms such as those recommended by the British Geriatrics Society (see Appendix B). Ultimately of greatest importance have been initiatives undertaken at the local level by health service management authorities, by hospital-based consultants in geriatric medicine and at times their colleagues in other clinical fields, and occasionally by benefactors from the private sector.

The role of individual geriatric consultants in fashioning change and development of their units was repeatedly apparent. Specific examples are noted earlier in this section as well as in chapters 4 and 6. A variety of explicit tactics were adopted to accomplish such ends. Recurring themes in this regard include the following:

1. Cultivating the concept of rehabilitation-oriented team care in which members of other disciplines decide and implement patient care plans conjointly with the physician on the geriatrics service.

2. Providing prompt and effective consultation on difficult patients on surgical and medical services, thus winning respect and support for geriatric medicine among previously skeptical peers in other specialties.

3. Developing and maintaining formal lines of communication with general practitioners, community nursing services, and social work services to facilitate the complex process of coordinating inpatient and community care of the frail elderly patient.

4. Serving on hospital management committees, as well as medical advisory committees to district and regional health authorities and national standard-setting and certifying committees (e.g.,

---

*Regional- and district-level management authorities, which have themselves evolved over time with reorganization of the NHS in 1974 and 1982, have ultimate responsibility for hospital planning, management, and staffing decisions, including those related to development of geriatrics services. They in turn look to professional advisory committees for guidance in development or modification of hospital and related services. Within the hospitals proper, consultant physicians have traditionally retained strong jurisdiction over how the beds allocated to their respective specialty are used. In 1985, in its quest for efficiency and accountability, the government issued a new organizational reform plan (the Griffiths Report) which calls for professional managers to assume primary responsibility for resource allocation in the NHS. Useful discussion of the evolving process of decision making and resource allocation in the NHS is found in Rudolph Klein's *The Politics of the National Health Service* (1983). A recent article entitled "Central Accountability and Local Decision-Making: Towards a New NHS" by Day and Klein (1985) considers the impact of the new, more centrally determined management of the NHS called for in the Griffiths Report.

General Medical Council, Joint Committee on Higher Medical Training, Hospital Advisory Service), to vigorously promote the needs of geriatric medicine for upgraded facilities, increased medical and remedial staff, and designated roles in undergraduate and postgraduate medical education.

The role of other specialties in developing geriatrics services was cited a number of times during the site visits. For instance, departments of medicine took the initiative to foster strong geriatrics services as an integral, but clearly designated (in terms of access to beds and house staff) component of general medicine. This was very apparent in the three "integrated" units visited: Great Yarmouth, Newcastle, and Oxford. In the last case, this strategy was implemented under the then Regius Professor of Medicine, Dr. Paul Beeson, who has subsequently played a vigorous role in promoting geriatric medicine in the United States (see ch. 10). (An illustrative "case study" of the unit at Great Yarmouth is provided in Appendix F.) Departments of orthopedic surgery, and in one instance urology (Cardiff), also initiated a variety of cooperative arrangements with geriatrics services to facilitate postoperative rehabilitation of elderly patients. Particularly exemplary in this regard were departments in Hastings, Edinburgh, Manchester, Glasgow, Nottingham, and Cardiff.

The role of regional and district management was most apparent in the form of resource development, as illustrated earlier in this chapter. Specific examples, reflecting complementary efforts between management and consultants include the following:

1. Decisions in the Oldham health district in the late 1970s to assign general medicine registrars and senior house officers to the geriatrics unit in response to a survey by the geriatric consultants demonstrating that the majority of their admissions had active medical as well as rehabilitation problems.
2. Decision by the management team for the South Glamorgan Health Authority (Cardiff) in 1982 to divert funds originally scheduled for opening three new medical intensive care beds to open instead eighteen geriatric rehabilitation beds, the need for which had been convincingly demonstrated by data furnished by the geriatrics department (personal communication, Dr. Deirdre Hine, community medicine specialist, March 1983).
3. Establishment of professorial departments of geriatric medicine in Edinburgh (1976) and Cardiff (1979). In both instances the importance of a strong academic presence in order to attract and train future geriatricians was vigorously promoted by geriatric consultants affiliated with the respective medical schools. The chief administrative medical officers for the respective regions in

turn negotiated the professorial posts and provision of beds, within teaching hospitals, to be financed from Health Service developmental funds.

Finally, the role of private benefactors in developing the field of geriatric medicine was noted. They have endowed professorial chairs at several medical schools (e.g., Birmingham, Glasgow, St. George's) and supported research facilities (e.g., Ciba-Geigy Unit for Research in Ageing, University of Manchester, Cargill Geriatric Research Unit at the University of Glasgow).

Summary

In one respect the "grande tour" of geriatrics departments fulfilled the words of Dr. James Williamson, who advised that "if you visit one hundred departments you will find one hundred different systems of care!" (personal communication, August 1981). Indeed, no two departments were the same with respect to the many details of staffing, resources, and day-to-day activity. Some in fact had evolved particularly unique approaches to certain aspects of providing geriatric care. However, when the twenty departments, located in widely varied settings, are compared from the perspective of providing an organized continuum of medical care for the vulnerable elderly, the similarities far overshadow the differences. The generic elements of such departments are well depicted in figure 5-2. Each serves a clearly defined population; provides a continuum of acute assessment, rehabilitation, respite, and long-term care services involving inpatient and day hospital facilities; maintains liaison with community

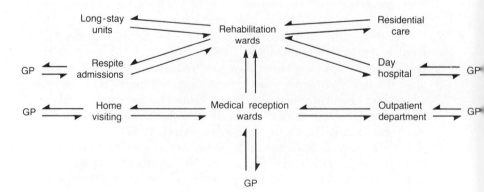

Figure 5-2 Basic elements of a hospital-based geriatric medicine unit.
Source: Adapted from Evans, J. G. 1983. Integration of geriatric with general medical services in Newcastle. *Lancet* 1:1430–33. Reprinted with permission.

medical (general practice), nursing, and social services and with selected other hospital-based departments; and is staffed by specialist consultants, medical house officers, nurses, social workers, and remedial therapists who work as a multidisciplinary team.

CHAPTER 6

The Impact of Geriatric Medicine
on Hospital Utilization

The inclusion of the geriatric unit in a general hospital, with all modern facilities and the necessary staff for investigation, consultation, and treatment, would raise the standard of work done, shorten the time of stay in hospital, and avoid the unnecessary blocking of beds by patients who could be treated sufficiently to return to their own homes or enter a home.

—M. W. WARREN, 1946

Efficient and effective use of hospital services by elderly persons is one of the overriding objectives and in some respects the raison d'être of organized geriatrics services. Historically this objective gave rise to the geriatrics movement in Great Britain and remains the focus in that country as well as in the United States and other nations seeking solutions to the burgeoning medical needs and costs of elderly persons. Therefore, this chapter specifically explores strategies adopted by geriatrics departments to use inpatient services effectively; where available, quantitative assessment of the strategies' impact on utilization is included. The chapter constitutes a summary of published and unpublished experiences among the twenty units visited, supplemented with related studies from elsewhere in Great Britain. Special attention is given to defining "bed blocking" and the roles played by geriatric medicine services in alleviating or preventing such occurrences.

As depicted in figure 6-1, geriatric medicine departments may affect hospital utilization by intervening at several different points in the continuum of services. These points include preventing admission to hospital from home or readmission from long-stay institutions, and expediting discharge of potential bed-blocking patients from hospital. Strategies that accomplish one or the other of these purposes are natural outgrowths of the structural and operational

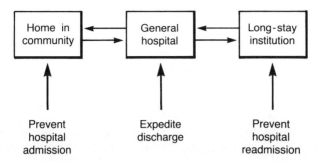

Figure 6-1 Points of intervention by geriatrics departments to reduce hospital utilization.

components of geriatrics departments discussed in the previous two chapters.

Prevention of Admission and Readmission

Prevention of hospital admission or readmission of elderly persons may be achieved through vigorous application of principles of geriatric medicine in caring for patients in their own homes or in continuing care institutions. In both instances, this involves close collaboration between a hospital-based geriatrics service and the patient's personal primary care physician and other support services.

Home in the Community

A common dilemma that may lead to hospitalization of elderly persons from their home arises when a partially disabled but medically stable elderly person who lives alone becomes temporarily incapacitated due to acute illness. Under these circumstances, the GP commonly refers the patient directly to a hospital-based specialist for hospitalization. As an alternative to such hospitalization, geriatrics departments may provide emergency home assessment and assistance in arranging short-term supportive nursing and social services in the community.

The value of such a strategy has been assessed in a pilot "augmented home care" project, developed by the University of Edinburgh Department of Geriatric Medicine. This project evolved from the observation that as many as 30 percent of acute hospitalizations of elderly patients from home could be prevented if short-term intensive community nursing and home help services were provided to supplement medical care provided by the patient's general practitioner (Currie, Smith, and Williamson 1979). In the pilot study such patients, most of whom experienced acute infections or cardiovascular events, were managed at home, and their medical outcomes proved comparable to those for a similar group who were hospitalized. Also, the patients managed at home required less time to recover their previous level of functioning in activities of daily living (Currie et al. 1980). A randomized controlled trial, including estimates of potential cost savings of the augmented home care scheme, was initiated in 1983–84. This project, with its favorable results in avoiding unnecessary hospitalization, is analogous to the widely recognized and highly successful randomized trial of home management of uncomplicated myocardial infarction reported by British investigators some years earlier (Mather et al. 1976).

Long-Stay Institutions

When patients residing in long-stay geriatric institutions develop acute illnesses that would ordinarily lead to admission to an acute hospital, it was found to be standard practice for such patients to be treated in the long-stay institution by a general practitioner or house officer attached to the geriatrics service. The necessary twenty-four-hour nursing care, including capacity to administer intravenous fluids or medications, was available in the long-stay setting, as was consultation with the district geriatrician as needed. An informal survey of the twenty geriatrics units I visited yielded estimated rates of 3–6 hospitalizations per 100 long-stay beds per year. This rate is less than one-fifth the rate of acute hospitalizations expected among the elderly. The few hospitalizations that did occur were for acute problems requiring sophisticated technical services of a general hospital (e.g., fractured femur, diabetic coma).

A special analysis of the routine admission and discharge statistics for 1984 of the City Hospital geriatrics department in Edinburgh revealed a total of 5 acute hospitalizations from 204 long-stay beds, or 2.5 per 100 beds. All 5 were occasioned by fracture of the femur (personal communication, Dr. James Williamson, October 1985). An accompanying prospective survey of all medically attended problems in one 90-bed long-stay institution in Edinburgh was conducted for the four-month period March–June of 1984. A total of 422 problems were documented, as shown in table 6-1. Forty-six (11 percent) of the episodes were attended on an urgent basis by a house officer from the acute geriatrics unit, while the rest were discussed and managed at routine medical-nursing conferences. One patient was transferred to the acute hospital for treatment of a fractured femur (personal communication, Ann Brayer, June 1986).

Table 6-1
Medically Attended Problems during a Three-Month Period in a Ninety-Bed
Long-Stay Geriatrics Facility in Edinburgh

Problem	Number	Percent
Urinary tract infection	42	10
Constipation	38	9
Fall	33	8
Agitation	22	5
Skin infection	21	5
Eye irritation, infection	17	4
Dyspnea, heart failure	15	4
Nausea, vomiting	15	4
Rash, itching	15	4
Lower respiratory infection	13	3
All other	191	44
TOTAL	422	

Source: Personal communication, A. Brayer, 1985.

The Bed-Blocking Problem

The blocking of acute medical and surgical beds by hospitalized elderly patients, alluded to as long ago as 1946 in Marjory Warren's writings, has continually posed a major challenge to British hospital services. Many case studies as well as community-wide hospital surveys have attempted to quantitate and understand this problem and recommend practical solutions. While some studies have used a hospital stay of greater than thirty days as an objective basis for defining bed blocking, such an arbitrary quantitative definition has been of limited value because it misclassifies both inappropriately long stays of less than thirty days and appropriate hospital stays of greater than thirty days duration. The following more flexible, albeit subjective definition was derived from a survey of British regional health authorities in 1976: "A blocked bed is a bed occupied by a patient who in the consultant's opinion no longer requires the services provided for that bed, but who cannot be discharged or transferred to more suitable accommodation" (Ashley, Laurence, and Hughes 1981, 3).

A selection of studies of the bed-blocking problem in a number of settings provides useful insight into the role of organized geriatrics services as part of the solution. A case study in 1968 examined the experiences of a number of individual disabled elderly patients whose physicians deemed them unsuitable to remain on acute medical or surgical inpatient services. A series of calamities befell these patients as they either languished in acute hospital beds or were discharged to the community, with little attention paid to rehabilitation or continuing care needs. Seeing these patients as victims of an outdated but lingering division between the delivery of acute and chronic care, the author cited one of the fundamental potential contributions of the NHS: "With the coming of the Health Service the dividing lines were redrawn and came to lie not between 'acute' and 'chronic' but between those who needed a home and those who needed a hospital" (Binks 1968, 271). He in turn discussed at some length the unsuitability of restricting the role of the general hospital to acute medical care, hence neglecting those in need of chronic and rehabilitative care who by definition become "bed blockers." In sum, "Our present battles are not going to be won using the last war's weapons, tactics, and strategy" (p. 273).

In a widely cited report with a somewhat different tone, an assessment of the bed-blocking situation in the general medical services of a large teaching hospital in Glasgow in the early 1970s concluded with the following statement: "The acute medical ward is unable to offer its highly specialized and expensive resources to the appropriate patients because one third of its beds are occupied by patients no longer in need of medical care" (McArdle, Wylie, and Alexander 1975, 569). This article elicited a lively series of letters, largely from geriatricians, calling for a broadening of the role of the general hospital and a greater presence of geriatric practices and resources within the acute hospital (Braverman 1975; Coni 1975).

Community-wide surveys of both surgical and medical inpatient services have further quantified and elucidated the bed-blocking problem. In a point prevalence survey of 1,010 occupied acute medical beds among three general hospitals in Liverpool, 48 (4.8 percent) elderly patients were judged to be in beds inappropriate to their needs. The investigators, representing both the health and social service departments of the Liverpool metropolitan area, examined the inpatient records of the 48 patients and found extensive evidence of poor management. Specifically, geriatric, social work, and rehabilitation consultation, which could have been very helpful, had been infrequent and usually not initiated until four weeks or more from the time of the patient's admission to hospital. Furthermore, on only one of the patients was a joint assessment and care plan performed by personnel from these several disciplines (Rubin and Davies 1975).

A one-day point prevalence survey of 325 surgical and orthopedic beds in one health district in London found 43 (13 percent) occupied inappropriately. The median age of the patients was 83. As in the Liverpool survey, review of records revealed a lack of timely or overall assessment of patient problems and long delays or total neglect of discharge planning. The author, a health authority medical officer, suggested that "rehabilitation advice to ward staff from a geriatrician" would be of much value in such cases, and that "shared care or combined ward rounds might be advantageous." Echoing other sentiments, he concluded with a general observation about prevailing attitudes that contribute to the bed-blocking problem: "It is all too easy to see the blocked bed problem as a misuse of expensive technology, whereas it is even more a dis-service to patients who are misplaced and lacking in the attention they need" (Murphy, 1977, 1396).*

Expediting Discharge

Reducing unnecessary prolongation of hospital stays has been the primary measurable impact of geriatrics services upon hospital utilization by the elderly. While the essential measure of impact has been overall length of hospital stay, impact has also been apparent in the form of reduction in numbers of bed-blocking elderly patients, on other hospital services, awaiting geriatric consultation or transfer. A series of published and unpublished case studies illustrates the effectiveness of various organizational strategies, both internal and external to geriatrics departments, in reducing hospital stays.

Internal Strategies

The geriatrics departments in both Hull (Bagnall et al. 1977) and Oldham (O'Brien, Joshi, and Warren 1973) have published detailed descriptive analyses of the impact of their age-related services upon various parameters of hospital utilization by the elderly. In both instances, the implementation of age-related services, channeling virtually all hospital referrals over age 65 in Oldham and over age 75 in Hull directly to geriatrics departments based in district general hospitals, resulted in the following:

1. Reduction in average length of stay of elderly persons admitted to hospital.
2. Elimination of bed-blocking elderly patients on general medical

---

*A further case in point is found in a recent report on bed blocking in the Bromley health district of the greater London area. A prevalence survey in 1983 revealed that over 10 percent of district hospital beds, particularly those in general medicine and orthopedic surgery, were occupied by "bed blockers." Historically, geriatric medicine was provided with few acute care hospital facilities in the district. In light of the survey findings, late in 1985 a decision was taken on the part of physicians in general medicine, who had previously adamantly rejected such proposals, to convert part of the general medicine service into an age-related (75 and over) acute geriatrics service. Preliminary follow-up in 1986 indicated reduction in the bed-blocking problem in the district (Coid and Crome 1986).

and surgical services awaiting transfer to geriatrics for rehabilitation or continuing care disposition.
3. Avoidance of hospital admission for many who would otherwise
have been admitted, by arranging for alternative provision of
medical as well as nursing, remedial, or social care in the community.

These experiences are at variance with those of other health districts, including ones proximate to Oldham and Hull, which experience sizable waiting lists of bed blockers on acute services and longer
average length of stay among hospitalized elderly. Such districts
have been less vigorous in allocating general hospital beds to geriatric medicine (Ashley, Laurence, and Hughes 1981). The success of
these two units and others like them in the United Kingdom (Das
Gupta 1980; Rai, Murphy, and Pluck 1985) is ascribed to advantages
realized by an age-related geriatrics unit that has early direct access
to most elderly patients referred to hospital and that in turn is based
predominantly in a general hospital, is well staffed with house officers, and has ready access to full diagnostic laboratory services
(Evans 1981).

An experience similar to that reported by the pioneering age-
related geriatrics departments in Oldham and Hull in the 1960s and
1970s was observed in the geriatric medicine department in the town
of Wrexham in North Wales. The department, which had formerly
operated a very active selective referral geriatrics service, evolved
into a partially age-related service late in 1982 with the conversion
of a twenty-bed general medicine ward to an acute admission geriatrics ward. This resource reallocation was decided by the hospital's
management committee with full support of the department of medicine, which had become frustrated with a chronic backlog of bed
blockers awaiting transfer to the geriatrics department. Over the
first ten months of operations of the acute geriatrics ward, beginning
in October 1982, the waiting list of bed-blocking elderly patients on
other services diminished from a previous monthly prevalence of 35–
40 down to 15–20 by February and less than 5 by August 1983.
Reasons for this phenomenon, in particular the vigorous application
of rehabilitation, are succinctly spelled out in a letter of 2 September
1983 from Dr. I. U. Shah, M.R.C.P., one of the geriatric consultants in
Wrexham:

> With regard to the activities on the part of the Geriatric Services [in
> Wrexham] the reasons which I believe have accounted for the decline in
> the size of the waiting list during 1983 are as follows.
> 1. The ability of the Geriatric Unit to offer a bed to patients in the
> community who require admission, instantly, means the institution

of rehabilitation at the earliest possible time. This definitely improves the success rate and consequently there is less demand on the long stay beds.

2. The transfer of care of elderly patients with acute medical problems from General Medicine to the Geriatric Unit with far superior and better organised rehabilitation facilities has resulted in marked reduction in the average length of stay of these patients in hospital.

3. The ability of the Department of Geriatric Medicine to offer help to the carers straight away enables the carers to take the patient home when patients are ready for discharge. The carers no longer feel helpless and they know that help will be available if and when returned.

4. The ability to transfer patients from other departments to our Unit quicker also means the institution of rehabilitation at a much earlier and more appropriate stage. This again improves the success rate.

5. In the absence of waiting lists we are able to do more preventive work in the community, we are getting more earlier referrals, and the majority of these cases can be treated as out-patients.

6. The improvements in the relationship with the local Social Services Department and other community-based support services has resulted in early discharge of the patients requiring residential accommodation.

The selective referral Department of Health Care of the Elderly at the University of Nottingham also documented a significant impact upon lists of elderly patients on the general medical service awaiting geriatric consultation. In this instance it was found that increasing the complement of senior medical house officers on the geriatric assessment wards expedited the care and discharge of patients admitted to the service. This in turn freed geriatric consultants to respond more rapidly to patients in the department of medicine who were on the waiting list for consultation and disposition. Between January 1981 and January 1983, the list of such waiting patients steadily declined from 86 to 23 (personal communication, Dr. John Bendall, August 1983).

Finally, the integrated service in Newcastle, which combines geriatrics and general medicine, has been found to operate far more efficiently than would be the case with two administratively separate departments. Such a strategy is particularly valuable in settings such as Newcastle, which have a relative paucity of district general hospital beds available for adult medical patients, old and young alike (Evans 1983). An analogous strategy implemented in North Staffordshire in 1983 has shown evidence of a reduced overall percentage of elderly patients requiring discharge to long-stay institutions. This success is attributed to such major changes as making geriatric assessment and rehabilitation more immediately available to all hospitalized elderly medical patients and upgrading the medical house staff coverage for geriatric rehabilitation patients (Dunn and Patel 1983).

External Strategies

In 1977 the City Hospital Department of Geriatric Medicine in Edinburgh implemented a strategy of attaching consultants in geriatric medicine to acute medical wards in the main university teaching hospital to provide routine consultation on newly admitted elderly patients. This strategy was partly in response to the department of medicine's growing problem of bed blocking by elderly disabled patients. Using historical controls from 1975–76 for comparison, an evaluative study showed a significant reduction in average length of stay from twenty-five to sixteen days for elderly women admitted for acute care, particularly for those above 80 years of age, following introduction of the consultation strategy in 1977–78. In the published report of this experience, the authors offered the following comments to explain the observed impact:

> We cannot define exactly the reasons for the improvement but suggest that the following factors are important: (1) obtaining a prompt and complete social report; (2) multidisciplinary assessment of the patient by the doctor, nurse, physiotherapist, occupational therapists, and, of course, the medical social workers; (3) the special interest and experience in the psychiatry of old age that the geriatric team was able to bring to the ward; (4) early planning of arrangements to facilitate return to the community; (5) familiarity of the geriatric medicine team with the local community resources and how to mobilize them; (6) the ability of the geriatric team to arrange directly for geriatric aftercare for the patients returned home or, in the case of patients who went outside the team catchment area, to negotiate this with other geriatric teams in the region. (7) Possibly the most important single factor was the ability of the geriatric medicine specialist to decide when it was safe and suitable for an individual old patient to be returned home once a certain degree of independence had been achieved. This ability arises out of experience and cannot be achieved in any other way. Another similar factor is the weekly review of each elderly patient, even those who seem to be "stuck." Under the previous system once a patient's name had gone on the long-term list and been categorized as a "bed-blocker," the incentive to go on seeking alternatives tended to slow down or disappear. (Burley et al. 1979, 92)

A second evaluation in Nottingham examined the impact of the introduction in 1978 of an eighteen-bed orthogeriatric rehabilitation unit. The unit was designed for consultants from orthopedics and geriatrics to share responsibility for the postoperative rehabilitation and medical care of elderly women hospitalized with fractured neck of the femur complicated by other disease or disability. Comparing the experience of such patients in 1977, prior to introducing this unit, with that in 1979 revealed a decline in average total length of hospital stay for acute and rehabilitative care from sixty-six to forty-eight days. This decline in turn freed up orthopedic beds to expedite admission of patients on waiting lists for elective surgery (Boyd et al. 1984). Formal evaluation of a similar arrangement between orthopedic surgery and geriatric medicine at the Whittington Hospital in London achieved an estimated 38 percent reduction in hospital bed days for elderly patients with hip fracture (personal communication, Dr. Patrick Murphy, March 1986). Such successes with joint orthopedic-geriatric units or consultative services were also reported during visits to the geriatrics units in Cardiff, Edinburgh, Hastings, and St. George's Hospital in London. A randomized clinical trial of such a unit was initiated by the University of Manchester Department of Geriatric Medicine in 1984.

Comment

The sum of these experiences indicate that organized geriatrics services have had significant impact on hospital utilization in a variety of situations. In seeking common denominators among particular experiences, several are apparent.

First is the essential factor of bringing the practice of geriatric medicine into the acute general hospital setting. This arrangement has occurred primarily through allocating general hospital beds directly to geriatric medicine, and secondarily through developing various consultative liaison activities with acute medical and surgical services. The critical importance of such organizational arrangements, while evident in the individual experiences discussed here, is further substantiated by analyses from the national perspective. In Ashley, Laurence, and Hughes's 1981 survey of some ninety health authorities, it was commonly reported that bed blocking was more severe in those districts lacking strong geriatrics services in the general hospital sector and less severe (in some instances absent) where the converse was the case. An analysis of national hospital statistics provides indirect quantitative evidence, showing that those districts with the most effective geriatrics services (including Hull and Oldham, described earlier) have 6–8 general hospital beds per

1,000 elderly persons compared with a national average of 3 (Evans 1981).

Given district general hospital beds with ready access to diagnostic services and the presence of house officers to meet patients' medical needs, the other essential characteristic common to successful geriatrics services is the infusion of geriatric rehabilitation and managerial principles. These are eloquently attested to in the words from the article by Burley et al. and in the letter from Dr. Shah cited earlier.

While this chapter has intentionally restricted its focus to hospitalization, this is only one, albeit particularly conspicuous and costly, component of the continuum of health care of the elderly. A short statement to this effect entitled "The Spectrum of Care," accompanied by a comprehensive chart depicting community as well as institutional components, was developed by Dr. James Williamson (1981) as part of a symposium on Appropriate Care for the Elderly convened in Scotland in 1980. This statement is reproduced in Appendix G and serves as a fitting transition from consideration of the hospital to consideration of the community component of services for the elderly.

CHAPTER 7

Care in the Community

Providing health care in the home or elsewhere in the community on an ambulatory basis in lieu of admission to institutions has long been a guiding philosophy in Great Britain. This philosophy has become increasingly central to health or related social service policies for the elderly as the size and cost of care for this particular vulnerable segment of population has grown in recent decades. Paralleling and complementing the developments of geriatric medicine in the hospital have been a variety of pragmatic and policy initiatives promoting primary medical care and social services for the elderly in the community.

Under the terms of the National Health Service Act (1946), virtually all persons are enrolled, by mutual consent, with a community-based general practitioner who is responsible for providing and coordinating their health care, including referral to hospital-based specialists. This arrangement, which emerged from the "referral system" negotiated by mutual consent between general practitioners and consultant physicians in the later part of the nineteenth century (Stevens 1966), has become central to the provision of comprehensive care for the elderly. Great Britain also has a long-standing tradition of providing nursing and social services in the home. Originating in large measure to meet the health care needs of expectant mothers and their newborns, the widespread deployment of visiting nurses, social workers, and home helps as part of public health and welfare reform early in the twentieth century established community-based resources of critical importance to current comprehensive approaches to care of the elderly (Nepean-Gubbins 1972; Connolly 1980). This chapter examines the contemporary functions of general practice, nursing, and social services provided for the community-dwelling elderly, with particular attention to the ways these various services are linked together and linked with hospital-based geriatric medicine departments, as shown schematically in figure 7-1.

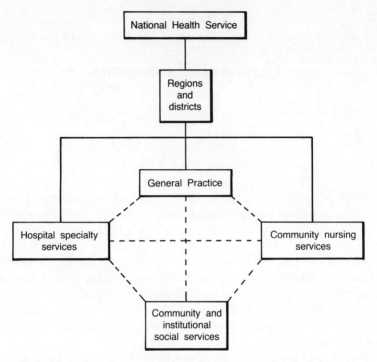

Figure 7-1 Basic components of organized health and social services in Great Britain.

Community Surveys

With the coming of the NHS, hospital boards concerned with project-ing and planning for future needs of elderly persons undertook com-munity surveys in a number of locales in Britain. Among the earliest and most renowned was a cross-sectional survey of a random sample of some 583 aged persons living in their own homes in the town of Wolverhampton, England, conducted under the sponsorship of the Nuffield Provincial Hospitals Trust. The resulting report, entitled *The Social Medicine of Old Age* (Sheldon 1948), described a full spec-trum of states of health in the elderly population, from those who were disease-free and totally independent, to those with significant mental and/or physical disabilities, often unattended by a doctor. Community surveys with similar findings were conducted in the ear-ly 1950s in Birmingham, Glasgow, and elsewhere (Armstrong 1983).

A later wave of surveys replicated these findings and recom-mended various innovative health services for the community-dwell-ing elderly. Exemplary among these was a study entitled "Old People at Home: Their Unreported Needs," conducted by a hospital-based geriatric medicine unit in Edinburgh (Williamson et al. 1964). This study was prompted by the authors' observations that elderly patients were often referred to the geriatric hospital unit at a very advanced stage of disease and disability. Their survey, involving a sample of some two hundred elderly patients enrolled with three different general practices, documented an average of three to four disabilities per person, over half of which were not known to their general practitioner. The majority of unattended problems consisted of disabilities with ambulation or micturation or one of two major mental health afflictions of old age, depression and dementia. The patients and their doctors frequently ascribed such problems to old age rather than illness and therefore tended to do little about them. The authors of this study and others, particularly in Scotland, recommended developing "preventive geriatrics" strategies whereby such disabilities might be actively sought out and brought to medical attention early for assessment and remedial intervention, rather than depending upon the traditional approach of self-reporting of medical problems by patients (Williamson, Lowther and Gray 1966; Anderson 1974).

They further suggested that general practitioners maintain a registry of their elderly patients to help assure periodic screening to detect changes in their health and social circumstances. Community nurses might undertake much of the responsibility for such health surveillance of the vulnerable elderly.

Various of these ideas were tested by geriatric medicine units, first in the Glasgow area (Anderson and Cowan 1955) and later in Edinburgh, through development of consultative clinics to which GPs might refer elderly patients for screening and assessment. In such a service, community nurses trained in assessing the elderly patient were found to be effective at detecting disabilities. Among 300 consecutive referrals, potentially remediable disabilities were found in 194, and the recommended therapy or management was carried out in 161. At follow-up, improvement was evident in half of those who carried out recommendations, and this improvement was attributable to earlier diagnosis than would have been achieved without these clinics in 42 percent of cases. The authors concluded that "the offer of a routine examination to high risk groups is of benefit to old people and a form of medical practice which should be widely adopted" (Lowther, MacLeod, and Williamson 1970, 275).

General Practice and Preventive Geriatrics

During the past decade, preventive geriatrics strategies have in fact been adopted as an integral component of general practice in many

parts of Great Britain. These developments, inspired by the earlier
work from geriatric medicine units, have been greatly facilitated by
several health policy initiatives with direct bearing on the delivery of
primary care in Great Britain. First, the Family Doctor Charter,
adopted by the NHS in 1965, amended terms of GP services to provide
subsidy for improving practice premises, record systems, and ancil-
lary staffing, and importantly, to provide supplemental stipends for
caring for elderly patients (British Medical Association 1965). Second, as part of a broad national policy commitment to fostering the
"health team" approach to delivering primary care, the Public
Health Services Act amendments of 1968 officially condoned and
encouraged the direct attachment of visiting nurses and other community health professionals to GP practices and health centers. Under this policy these personnel could be shifted from their traditional
commitments of serving patients within a defined geographical area
to instead serving solely those patients enrolled in one or more general practices to which the health professionals are administratively
"attached" (Reedy 1979). Third, a major administrative reorganization of the National Health Service in 1974 (enacted two years earlier
in Scotland), with the intent of improving coordination between hospital specialities, general practice, and community health services,
created important formal liaisons, particularly between GPs and
hospital consultants (Zwick 1985).

Under these circumstances, preventive strategies, such as those
originally fostered by geriatric medicine departments, became more
fully incorporated into the primary care domain. Rather than refer
elderly patients to screening clinics organized by geriatrics departments, which could accommodate only limited numbers of patients,
progressive general practitioners developed health screening and
surveillance strategies within their practice operations. The essential ingredients for such an activity included an age-sex register for
easy identification of elderly patients in the practice, a practical
method for systematically inquiring into a person's possible unmet
health or social needs, and one or more practice-attached visiting
nurses to carry out the health surveillance. Positive findings from the
nurse's assessment would result in arranging for the GP to follow up
on medical problems that were detected or for the area social work
office or other community-based services to follow up on social needs.

Several studies have evaluated the effectiveness and efficiency of
these practice-based programs. A randomized trial involving a general practice in Oxford found that those elderly patients for whom a
nurse-operated program of health surveillance was provided utilized
approximately 30 percent fewer hospital days (288 versus 407 per 100
persons per year) and showed less frequent decline in functional

independence over a two-year period. Among the 145 patients in the surveillance group, 144 medical conditions (primarily circulatory, musculoskeletal, and neurological) were newly detected, some half of which improved with specific intervention. This group also received significantly more referrals for short- and long-term community-based social support services in comparison with the control group (Tullock and Moore 1979). In a quasi-experimental evaluation of a similar practice-based assessment program in Glasgow, a cohort of 100 elderly patients was found to have marked reduction in unmet health and social needs on reassessment some six to twelve months after an initial assessment had been performed. Table 7-1, adapted from data in this study, shows the magnitude of improvement in service delivery for unattended symptomatology that occurred presumably as a result of the assessment program (Barber and Wallis

Table 7-1
Health and Health Service Delivery Benefits from Geriatric Assessment Program in a Glasgow General Practice

Medical Categories	Number Requiring Action	
	First Assessment	Second Assessment
General health	8	10
Gastrointestinal	16	5
Skin	4	3
Genitourinary tract	10	7
Locomotor	6	2
Cardiorespiratory	15	11
Nervous system	11	5
Memory	5	1
Depression	16	7
TOTAL	91	51

Service Categories	Number with Unmet Service Needs	
	First Assessment	Second Assessment
Chiropody	21	4
Home help	16	4
Meals-on-wheels	3	6
Contacts	14	4
Housing	18	16
Nursing services	—	3
Supportive visits	47	1
Others	22	18
TOTAL	141	56

Source: Adapted from Barber and Wallis 1978. Reprinted with permission.
Note: n = 100 patients.

1978). A more recent randomized trial examined the effects of annual health assessment and referral by practice-attached visiting nurses in both urban and rural settings in Wales. In the urban practice, there was significant reduction in mortality and increase in sense of well-being among recipients of the special program while no differences were observed between experimental and control groups in the rural practice (Vetter, Jones, and Victor 1984).

In addition to these several evaluations of outcomes of preventive geriatrics strategies in general practice, a number of authors have reported a significant impact on process of primary care of the elderly in the form of reduced workload. One practitioner who kept account of the practice hours per week devoted to his elderly patients found these hours decreased somewhat following introduction of a periodic health and social assessment provided by himself and a practice-attached nurse. In explanation he offered the comment that "the time-gain is easily seen when one considers patients and relatives who are reassured, less isolated and less insecure and whose problems have been sorted out long before they have become a demanding, traumatic confrontation at weekends or other inconvenient times" (Hay 1976, 447). A second practitioner noted that after several years of a program of geriatric screening and supportive interventions, the annual rate of medical contacts of elderly persons in his practice was as much as 20 percent lower than the national average (Pike 1976). In a carefully quantitated study, Barber and colleagues determined that an initial investment of time to plan and conduct their geriatric screening program resulted not only in improved health outcomes for the patients, as discussed in the previous paragraph, but also in reduced workload for both general practitioners and practice-attached community nurses (Barber and Wallis 1982).

General Practice Surveys in Edinburgh

The considerable extent to which the practice of preventive geriatrics and related services for elderly patients have become part of primary care in Great Britain is indicated in findings from a survey of general practices in the Lothian Health Board area, which encompasses metropolitan Edinburgh and surrounding townships. (See Appendix A for methods and survey instrument.) A 25 percent representative sample of some 450 GPs practicing in the Lothian area were surveyed, and responses were received from 91 (81 percent response rate). Approximately 75 percent worked in partnerships with 2–5 other GPs, while the other respondents were evenly divided between solo practices or large partnership practices. Median practice population size was 1,708, with 242 (14.2 percent) persons over age 65, 105 (6.2 percent) of whom were over age 75.

Table 7-2 indicates the high degree to which age-sex registers, attached community nurses (district nurses and health visitors), and routine nurse surveillance of high-risk elderly have become part of general practice. These arrangements were reported for all sizes of practice, though they were somewhat more common among those GPs working in partnerships of three or more. Part-time attachments of chiropodists, physical therapists, occupational therapists, and social workers were reported in smaller percentages, primarily from the large practice arrangements where sufficient numbers of patients would merit locating such referral services within the practice premises.

The survey also found that virtually all respondents make house calls to frail elderly patients (median of 6–10 per week); make selective referrals to hospital-based geriatric medicine services (median of 6–10 patients per year); and provide primary care for elderly patients in nursing homes or long-term residential facilities (median of 6–10 patients). Rates of all of these activities tended to be higher for those GPs carrying disproportionately large numbers of persons over age 75 in their practice.

Further definition of the spectrum and content of primary care of the elderly is provided from a detailed survey of a full year's experience of the elderly members of one four-man general practice in Edinburgh. Each GP carried a population of approximately 1,800 persons, of whom 17–18 percent were over age 65. The practice included two attached community nurses (one health visitor and one district nurse) who conducted regular health surveillance of high-

Table 7-2

The Number and Percentage of General Practices with Selected Support Systems and Services for Community Care of the Elderly in Lothian Health District, Scotland

Support Systems and Services	Number	Percent
Age-sex register	58	64
Attached district nurse(s)	73	80
Attached health visitor(s)	69	76
Surveillance of "high-risk" elderly	61	67
Part-time physiotherapist	24	26
Part-time chiropodist	23	25
Part-time occupational therapist	8	9
Part-time social worker	7	8

Note: n = 91 practices.

risk elderly patients in their home, with the help of an age-sex register.

A retrospective review of medical and nursing records was conducted for calendar year 1982, utilizing a 20 percent systematic sample of elderly persons (every fifth patient over age 65 in the age-sex register). Indexes of general health status showed 43 percent and 15 percent of the younger (65 to 74 years old) and older (75 and above) groups to be "healthy" (i.e., no evidence of active chronic disease), with 3 percent of the former and 10 percent of the latter expiring during the year. Major chronic problems in virtually all domains were markedly more common among those aged 75 or above, with miscellaneous disabilities, ophthalmic, orthopedic, and mental problems being treated two to four times as often in this age-group (table 7-3). Approximately 90 percent of persons in both 65–74 year-old and 75+ year-old age-groups had one or more direct contacts with their GP; 35 percent of the former and 45 percent of the latter were referred to hospital-based specialists one or more times; and 33 percent of the 75+ group received one or more services from community nurses compared with only 6 percent of the 65–74 year-old group. Rates and reasons for contacts with a GP and referral to hospital specialists are shown in tables 7-4 and 7-5. The older group had an average of 7.2 GP contacts per person versus 5.2 for the younger group, with distributions according to primary reason for contact being similar. Both age-groups had approximately 1 specialty referral per 10 GP contacts, giving rates of 73 and 52 referrals per 100 persons per year, respectively. Reasons for specialty referral were

Table 7-3

Indexes of Health Status among a Sample of Elderly Persons in a General Practice in Edinburgh, 1982

Indexes of Health	65–74 Y/O (n = 117)		75+ Y/O (n = 105)	
	No.	Percent	No.	Percent
"Healthy"	50	43	16	15
One or more chronic conditions	63	54	78	75
Deaths	4	3	11	10
Chronic problems				
Heart, lung	42	36	58	55
Miscellaneous disabilities	7	6	34	32
Ophthalmic	9	8	24	23
Orthopaedic	10	9	19	18
Mental	6	5	20	19
Dermatologic	5	4	2	2
Miscellaneous organs	25	21	18	17

Table 7-4
The Number of Direct Contacts with a General Practitioner per Person among a
Sample of Elderly Persons in a General Practice in Edinburgh, 1982

	Contacts per 100	
	65–74 Y/O (n = 117)	75+ Y/O (n = 105)
All contacts	5.2	7.2
Active symptoms	2.1	2.9
Chronic care	1.7	2.2
Drugs only	1.2	1.8
Psychosocial	.2	.3

Table 7-5
The Number of Referrals to Hospital Specialists (Consultants) among a Sample of
Elderly Persons in a General Practice in Edinburgh, 1982

	Referrals per 100	
	65–74 Y/O (n = 117)	75+ Y/O (n = 105)
Reason for referrals		
Diagnostic advice	28	46
Hospital admission	12	20
Follow-up care	12	7
Total	52	73
By specialty		
General medicine	3	9
General surgery	5	7
Ophthalmology	5	7
Geriatrics	1	10
Pulmonary	3	7
GU/Gyn	3	5
ENT	3	5
Orthopedics	3	4
All others	26	19

again similarly distributed between the two groups, except that referrals to geriatric medicine were virtually all confined to the older age-group. The broad array of services both directly provided or arranged by community nurses for one or more patients during the year are listed in table 7-6.

General Practitioners and Geriatrics

In addition to their fundamental role as primary care providers to the elderly in the community, as reviewed above, general practitioners in many instances play important roles in part-time appointments as

Table 7-6
Services Provided/Arranged by Community Nurses among a Sample of Elderly
Persons in a General Practice in Edinburgh, 1982

Nursing Care	Social and Environmental
Bathing	Home helps
Bowel care	Meals-on-wheels
Incontinence pads	Heating, plumbing
Walking aids	Phone installation
Dressing leg ulcers	Gardening aid
Dietary counseling	Attendance allowance
Bereavement counseling	Day care referral
Chiropody referral	Sheltered housing
Optician referral	Nursing home

clinical assistants (see fig. 8-1) in geriatrics units. In such capacity in day hospitals, inpatient assessment and rehabilitation units, or long-stay facilities, general practitioners working in concert with geriatricians provide ongoing primary medical care and assist in the medical component of multidisciplinary care of geriatric patients. This mutually compatible relationship between the two branches of medical practice has proved an invaluable supplement to the limited number of medical personnel formally trained in geriatrics and has additionally contributed to building linkages between hospital and community components of the Health Service as called for in the 1974 NHS reorganization. Published accounts by general practitioners involved in appointments in geriatrics units attest to the attractiveness and success of such arrangements (Courtney 1973; Buckley 1977).

The general practitioners' need for knowledge regarding the special mix of health and health-related problems of old age and their management has been addressed through joint efforts by the British Geriatrics Society and the Royal College of General Practitioners (1978), through the publication of several books (Wilcock, Gray, and Pritchard 1982; Thompson 1984), and through the sponsoring of short postgraduate courses (e.g., as described in ch. 4).

Community Social Services

The effective provision of rehabilitative and preventive strategies on the part of geriatric medicine departments and general practice, respectively, is dependent upon strong and evolving community nursing and social services. Important in this regard, the provision of community support services has been repeatedly emphasized in surveys and policies related to the elderly in Britain (Great Britain,

Department of Health and Social Security [DHSS] 1976, 1981a;
Zwick 1985). Underlying the emphasis on care in the community
have been the dual concerns both to provide for the greatest hap-
piness of old people and to avoid costly institutional care. A corollary
to these concerns has been recognition of the crucial role of family
care givers and the desire to support their efforts with formal assistance while not undercutting or displacing them (Jones and Vetter
1985).

The roles of community nurses as an integral part of hospital and
primary medical care for the elderly have been discussed and illustrated earlier in this chapter and in previous chapters. A comprehensive review of social services for the elderly is beyond the scope of this
book.* Rather, attention is given to the evolution of policies and
practices conducive to provision of organized social support services
in conjunction with health services in the community.

Sheldon's 1948 report, *The Social Medicine of Old Age,* in addition
to describing the diseases and disabilities among community-dwelling elderly persons, also notes the heavy burden of care often borne
by families, particularly the female members. In response to this
observation, the author recommended, "we must do everything possible to assist the family in the care of its aged dependents without at
the same time relieving it of the necessity for still taking an interest
in the matter" (p. 166). He specifically called for the establishment of
a national domestic help service to assist families in maintaining
disabled elderly members in their homes. While not undertaking to
create such a service on a national scale, the National Health Service
Act identified such needs and delegated to local government the responsibility for providing home help services. In spite of this early
recognition of needs, the 1950s saw relatively little development of
such community support services. There was in fact considerable
debate among medical professionals, social workers, and policy
makers regarding the wisdom of such provisions for fear that these
might lead family members to abandon their filial duty to care for
their elders (Means and Smiths 1985, ch. 6). This perception was
convincingly dispelled by a number of local studies of roles played by
families of patients referred to geriatrics departments (Exton-Smith
1952; Isaacs and Thompson 1960; Lowther and Williamson 1966) as
well as by a national survey, *The Aged in the Welfare State* (Townsend
and Wedderburn 1965).

In all of these instances, family members were found to play significant and essential roles, while, as noted in the following summary

*An excellent overall review of social services for the elderly in Great Britain may
be found in Tinker 1981.

84 Adding Life to Years

statement from Townsend and Wedderburn's survey, those limited services introduced under the National Assistance Act (the authorizing legislation for social services, as is the NHS Act for health services) played a further essential role: "The health and welfare services for the aged, as presently developing, are a necessary concomitant of social organization, and therefore, possibly of economic growth. The services do not undermine self-help, because they are concentrated overwhelmingly among those who have neither the capacities nor the resources to undertake the relevant functions alone. Nor, broadly, do the services conflict with the interests of the family as a social institution, because either they tend to reach people who lack a family or whose family resources are slender, or they provide specialised services the family is not equipped or qualified to undertake" (1965, 129).

In the 1950s, various reviews of the NHS emphasized the particular importance of community social support as an adjunct to the efficient operation of the hospital services. These studies specifically identified the role to be played by increasing the provision of home help services for elderly persons. Similar arguments were made by Lord Amulree, one of the founders of the British Geriatrics Society, and others in Parliament. They argued that the government should assume responsibility for providing meals-on-wheels and other in-home services for disabled elderly (Means and Smith 1985, ch. 6). It was apparent that these and various other support services exceeded the capacity of local voluntary organizations in which they had originally been vested. An amendment to the National Assistance Act in 1962 empowered and encouraged local government to provide meals, chiropody, and a variety of social and recreational services all designed to support elderly persons and their care givers in the community. In the absence of a national program such as the NHS to finance and implement these activities, there was much variation in effort among local governments. To better assure the provision of such services, the local authority Social Service Act was legislated in 1970. This created social service departments to coordinate the many community services legislated in the preceding decade. Such agencies are now found in virtually all communities in Great Britain, with local offices operating roughly parallel with district health services. The array of social assistance and direct services available to the community-dwelling elderly and their families includes various forms of supplemental finances, day care centers, respite or holiday relief, laundry service for patients with urinary incontinence, telephone and alarm services, domiciliary physical therapy, adoptive aides and devices to assist with activities of daily living, meals-on-wheels, and, of foremost importance, home helps (Gatherer 1981).

Effective integration of these social services for the elderly with the separately financed and separately administered health services has posed a continuing challenge. Toward this end, two related initiatives emerged from NHS policy making during the 1970s. The first was the creation, under the 1974 NHS Reorganization Act, of Joint Consultative Committees to facilitate the greater integration of hospital, general practice, community nursing, and community social services at the local level. While these committees brought representatives of the respective provider groups together for fact-finding and planning purposes, they made little impact in the absence of shared financial resources. This shortcoming was addressed by the second initiative, the so-called Joint Financing scheme (enacted by Parliament in 1976), whereby social service expenditures that helped relieve pressure on the health services could be financed from health service funds (Norton 1981).

This climate has spawned numerous innovative approaches to improving the provision of supportive services in the community. Lack of a clear direction or centrally prescribed policy to guide this exploratory activity is apparent on surveying the recent literature. One finds, as with the earlier experience of the geriatric medicine movement, much resourcefulness in developing community services in response to old people's needs and local opportunity. Illustrative of this resourcefulness was a symposium on Innovations in the Care of the Elderly, which included case reports on extended home help, domiciliary physiotherapy, a continence advisory service, a day center for the mentally impaired, and a number of other recently developed or refurbished social and/or health services—all developed within the Birmingham–West Midlands area. The services draw largely on existing resources and have as a common denominator the enhancement of quality and duration of noninstitutional life for disabled elderly persons (Isaacs and Evers 1984). Several recent policy analysis monographs document other current undertakings in community care from many parts of the country (DHSS 1981, 1983; Allen 1983).

Evaluation of the impact of community social services on enhancing quality of life, reducing requirements for long-term institutional care, and cutting down on public costs of caring for the elderly has been an important but elusive goal. In an extensive review of the state of the art of community care for the elderly, Johnson and Challis (1983) note a number of descriptive-analytic studies of individual projects, most of which report evidence of improved well-being among recipients of the specific service being studied. Regarding reduced institutionalization and cost, two carefully documented studies of intensive or augmented use of the home help service have reported significant impact, respectively, in preventing acute hospitalization (Currie et al. 1980) and long-term institutional care (Gibbins et al. 1982). The Kent Community Care Project has rigorously evaluated an imaginative strategy in which specifically trained social workers serve as "case managers" for severely disabled community-dwelling individuals. Working with a fixed budget of two-thirds the estimated cost for residential care, the case managers organize a mix of appropriate formal and informal services to meet the client's needs and avoid institutionalization. Results to date in this controlled experiment have shown significant enhancement of quality of life, reduction in mortality, and reduction in institutionalization among the experimental group (Davies and Challis 1980). An interesting study in progress is attempting to correlate intensity of social service provision within defined geographic areas with hospital utilization (admission rate, average length of stay) for several major medical conditions for which community social services are thought to play an important role in reducing the need for acute hospital care. Preliminary analyses have shown a significant correlation between community provision of social services and reduced average length of stay for women hospitalized for stroke (Schweitzer and Greenberg 1984).

Summary

The needs of elderly persons for primary care services that include health surveillance, preventive intervention, and social support have been well defined in community surveys in Great Britain since the late 1940s. These needs have in turn been addressed through a variety of practical innovations in delivery of primary medical care, in particular the forging of close working relationships between community nursing and general practice. Also, social services, many of which were originally developed to provide support for mothers and infants in the home (in particular the home help service), have been increasingly adapted to support dependent elderly persons living in the community. As is the case with hospital-based geriatrics services discussed in chapters 3 through 6, innovative developments in community-based services, including integration of the various elements as shown in figure 7-1, have been encouraged and facilitated by the existence of a comprehensive National Health Service and health policies that give priority to services for the elderly.

CHAPTER 8

Medical School and Specialty Training in Geriatrics

There is much to recommend geriatrics as a specialty comparable to paediatrics. The creation of such a specialty would stimulate those with a leaning to this type of work and raise the standard of the work done. This branch of medicine forms an important subject for the teaching of medical students and should form part of their curriculum.

—M. W. WARREN, 1946

As foreseen in Dr. Warren's prophetic statement quoted above, the development of specialty career opportunities as well as formal undergraduate medical education in geriatric medicine have indeed occurred as natural and necessary parts of the evolution of organized geriatrics services in Great Britain. Today, some forty years later, with approximately five hundred consultant positions located in district and teaching hospitals throughout the country, geriatric medicine has become one of the largest and the fastest-growing of the hospital specialties in Great Britain. Academic departments with professorial chairs have been established in half of the country's medical schools, and geriatrics is a required part of the curriculum in all but two medical schools. This chapter reviews the status of these career and curricular developments, noting in particular their close correspondence with the development of health and health-related services for the elderly delineated in previous chapters.

Medical Career Development

The current pattern of medical education and career development in Great Britain is depicted in figure 8-1. Standards for medical school curriculum and for qualifying as a medical school graduate are established by the General Medical Council, a body whose role is comparable to that of the Liaison Committee on Medical Education

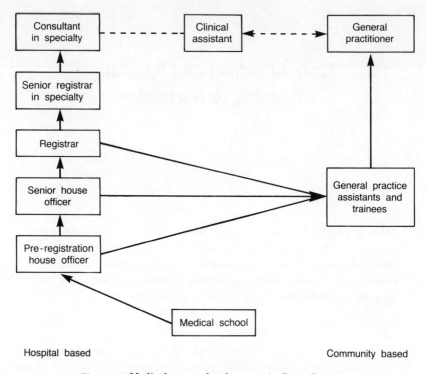

Figure 8-1 Medical career development in Great Britain.

(LCME) in the United States. (The LCME represents the American Association of Medical Colleges and the American Medical Association.)

Following five years in medical school (two preclinical, three clinical), all graduates spend a minimum of one year as a preregistration general house officer, rotating through medicine, surgery, and pediatrics. Then one generally pursues postgraduate training toward one of three fundamentally different medical careers: consultant in a hospital-based specialty (including geriatric medicine), general practitioner, or community medicine specialist. Those training for a hospital-based specialty spend one to three years as a senior house officer, followed by one or more years as a registrar on hospital services pertinent to the future field of specialization. (These positions are roughly analogous to the positions of assistant resident and chief resident, respectively, in the United States.) During this period, and prior to embarking on higher-level specialty training, the trainee must successfully pass a general specialty qualifying exam offered by the appropriate official academic society. Those planning to pursue higher training in geriatric medicine take the general medicine exam administered by the Royal College of Physicians and on successful completion are accorded Membership in the Royal College of Physicians—the MRCP. (This process is analogous to becoming board certified by the American Board of Internal Medicine in the United States.) The final stage of training prior to applying for a job as hospital consultant is that of senior registrar. This position, usually of two to four years duration, is analogous to a fellowship in a medical subspecialty in the United States and provides the candidate with a variety of educational, research, and practice activities related to the specialty. Educational standards to be met in senior registrar training programs for a given specialty (e.g., geriatric medicine) are established by the Joint Committee on Higher Medical Training, a standard-setting body that works closely with the academic specialty societies. On completing adequate training as a senior registrar, one applies for currently available consultant positions in one's specialty. Such consultantships are established by the individual regions of the National Health Service, in accordance with identified need in their hospital sector and availability of health service funds.

Candidates for careers in general practice or community medicine follow courses of training established by the designated academic societies in their respective specialties. All physicians working within the National Health Service (there is a small element of private practice in the country) are paid on a contract basis, with terms of employment and reimbursement negotiated between the central government and special standing committees of the British Medical Association which represent the various major subgroups within the medical profession.

Geriatrics in Medical School

In 1965 the University of Glasgow established the first medical school professorship and academic department of geriatric medicine in Great Britain, and in fact in the world. During its first decade the department developed a required curriculum for the clinical years of medical school which included three basic elements: a series of seminars on clinical problems and health services of particular importance to the elderly patient; supervised instruction in medical assessment of elderly patients on an acute geriatric inpatient unit, with emphasis on rehabilitative as well as acute care; and a series of home visits to elderly persons, which are designed to provide insight into the roles of general practitioners and nurses in caring for such patients in the community (Anderson 1976).

With growing awareness of the importance of health care of the elderly, manifest by the increasing presence of geriatric medicine units in general hospitals, the Glasgow experience in developing explicit curriculum for medical students was emulated elsewhere. This movement was strongly supported by a report on care of the elderly issued by the British Medical Association, which recommended that each medical school establish an academic unit "to provide authoritive undergraduate and postgraduate teaching in clinical problems of old people, together with some knowledge of gerontology and of the structure of services for the aged" (1976, 42). In 1980 the General Medical Council, in its "Recommendation on Basic Medical Education," called for all students to receive instruction in the special problems of diagnosis and treatment of illness in the elderly and in maintaining mental and physical health in old age. Instruction should also include introduction to the range of domiciliary and institutional services available for care of the elderly (1980).

A questionnaire survey sent to deans of all clinical medical schools in 1981 revealed, as noted earlier, that formal curriculum in geriatric medicine existed in 28 (93 percent) of the 30 schools, with academic departments of geriatric medicine in 14. Total required course time ranged from 3 to 171 hours, with a mean of 69 hours. Most teaching occurred during the clinical years and consisted of some combination of classroom and direct clinical instruction. Geriatric medicine was taught as a separate discipline in some schools, integrated into community care modules with general practice and community health in others, or taught in association with general medicine or psychiatry (Smith and Williams 1983).

A number of exemplary undergraduate teaching programs as well as a set of broad guidelines for teaching gerontology and geriatric medicine have been published in two special issues of *Age and Ageing,* the official journal of the British Geriatrics Society (Brocklehurst 1983; Stout 1985). In one particularly interesting report from the Welsh National Medical School in Cardiff, the effect of explicit educational experience in geriatrics was evaluated by randomly assigning medical students to clinical rotations on either the geriatric medicine or general medicine service. In a follow-up survey, students who were assigned to the geriatrics service were significantly more likely to hold favorable attitudes toward care of the elderly and to feel adequately prepared to manage medical problems in frail elderly patients, and were more disposed to consider a hospital career in geriatrics (Peach and Pathy 1982).

In seeking consensus on the essential ingredients of geriatric education for medical students, the World Health Organization sponsored a workshop in Edinburgh in 1982, drawing heavily on the collective experience in Great Britain (Stout 1985). Of fundamental importance in defining the field of geriatric medicine, both in the list of teaching objectives developed at this workshop and in the general statements from the British Medical Association and General Medical Council cited previously, is the emphasis on the health services as well as the biomedical aspects pertinent to medical care of the elderly.

Specialty Training

In 1946 when the National Health Service Act was legislated, there were four consultant physicians specializing in care of the elderly in Great Britain. With the NHS commitment to foster comprehensive medical services for the elderly, hospital consultant posts in geriatric medicine increased to over 100 by the early 1960s. This trend accelerated in the decade 1966–77, during which the number increased by 124 percent from 156 to 349. By contrast, the rate of increase in all hospital specialty positions during this time was 37 percent (Hutt, Parsons, and Pearson 1981). By 1985 the number of consultants in geriatric medicine was approximately 500, making geriatrics one of the largest clinical specialties in Great Britain. The growth in number of consultant positions is mirrored by that of senior registrar training positions. The first few of the latter were created in the early 1960s, with the number approaching 50 by 1970, 90 by 1980, and over 100 by 1984 (Brocklehurst 1984).

The very rapid growth in consultantships and training positions has posed significant challenges for the specialty of geriatric medicine. First has been the imperative to define the essential professional attributes of the specialty and develop standards for graduate training programs. Second has been the recruitment of medical graduates to such a rapidly expanding and nontraditional specialty.

From its inception in the 1940s, geriatric medicine has been broadly defined by its adherents as that field of medicine concerned with the curative, preventive, remedial, and social aspects of health and disease in the elderly. Following an initial period of largely pragmatic implementation of these principles on the part of its early leaders (see ch. 3), the specialty has been the subject of considerable effort at formal definition on the part of professional organizations vested with the authority to recommend and establish standards for medical training.

Among the earliest of such efforts was "Care of the Elderly in Scotland," a report produced under the auspices of the Royal College of Physicians of Edinburgh (1963). The report identified the need to establish hospital training positions at the senior registrar level in geriatric medicine to allow the future consultant to directly study the problems of the disabled elderly and work within the array of related health services. A follow-up report in 1970 noted that a substantial number of such positions for formal training of consultants in geriatrics had been established in Scottish health districts (Royal College of Physicians of Edinburgh 1970).

A committee on geriatric medicine established by the Royal College of Physicians of London in 1967 reached similar conclusions. In a report produced in 1972, the committee articulated a number of specific attributes of the specialty. With respect to clinical practice, the following were noted to be particularly important:

1. *Accurate Diagnosis.* The prognosis on which an elderly patient's future can be planned depends on accurate diagnosis. Common medical problems of the elderly are the coexistence of many disorders of disease and the predominance of vascular, neoplastic and degenerative conditions and nutritional deficiency. Diseases which also occur in younger patients may be modified by increasing age, or obscured by other conditions.
2. *Disability.* Disability has to be recognized as a factor in geriatric illness which merits assessment and treatment distinct from the disease processes which may underlie it.
3. *Mental Capacity.* It is essential to assess mental capacity (especially understanding, initiative, and willingness) as a factor affecting the prospects of elderly patients.
4. *Social Background.* The complex part played by environmental and other social factors is often of overriding importance in geriatric medicine. People usually retire at 65 and enter a phase of life when social factors become increasingly important and relatives and friends are also older and less able to help if illness develops. (P. 3)

Essential nonclinical attributes were also described:

In an ageing population the geriatric physician, though primarily based in the hospital, needs to be in close touch with those providing social and medical services for the community of which the elderly are a part. The geriatric physician expects to use his medical and managerial expertise as a member of a multidisciplinary team. He may also play an important part in research into the problems of ageing. (P. 2)

On the basis of such efforts from the Royal Colleges, the Joint Committee on Higher Medical Training, in consultation with the British Geriatrics Society, had by the later 1970s spelled out standards to be met in graduate training programs. Following three years as a house officer in general medicine, the candidate would spend four years of higher-level training. These might include rotations in various related specialties (e.g., neurology, psychiatry, cardiology) and/or laboratory research, plus two full years as senior registrar in a department of geriatric medicine. Specific to the senior registrar component, the JCHMT standards state: "Approved training posts, in Departments of Geriatric Medicine, include responsibility for the care of patients in acute, rehabilitation and continuing care units, day hospital and outpatient clinic and experience with assessment of patients at home. Specific training in administrative aspects of geriatric medicine is also required and psychogeriatric experience is especially desirable" (1980, 33).

Recruitment of physicians to fill traineeships and consultantships in geriatrics has proved problematic in the past, with fewer qualified candidates applying for posts, compared with applicants for other specialties, and a number of positions regularly going unfilled (DHSS, 1981).

A survey on determinants of doctors' career decisions was commissioned in 1976 by the Department of Health and Social Security (England and Wales) and the Scottish Home and Health Department to provide information that might guide policies for recruiting more candidates into several shortage specialties, including geriatrics. Among all doctors surveyed, it was found that most preferred treating acute disease and effecting cures and that very few liked dealing with social problems and health maintenance or predominantly with older patients. The majority had received no formal exposure to geriatrics in medical school. Of those surveyed who were practicing geriatric medicine, few had chosen this field prior to graduating from medical school; many had chosen to pursue a career in geriatrics some five to ten years later. A disproportionate number of this group were graduates of medical schools outside of Great Britain (Hutt, Parsons, and Pearson 1981).

These kinds of observations, along with a special report issued by a Working Party of the Royal College of Physicians of London (1977), lead to government initiatives encouraging the creation of consultant appointments in general medicine with special responsibility for the elderly (DHSS 1979). Such positions would be based in integrated departments in a general hospital (see chs. 3 and 5) in which the consultant would share acute care responsibilities for all types of medical patients with consultants in other medical specialities, while devoting a designated amount of time to rehabilitation and continuing care of elderly patients admitted to the service.

Such arrangements, which require close cooperation between existing general medicine and geriatrics services, have been developed in some health districts in England (though less so in Scotland) and appear, in terms of average number of applicants per job, to be slightly more popular than straight geriatric medicine posts (Graham and Playfair 1983).

Consultant Survey

As one means of defining the state of development of the specialty of geriatrics in Great Britain, Barker and Williamson conducted a survey of recently appointed consultants in 1983. (A copy of the survey instrument with explanatory narrative is contained in Appendix A.) The findings, as briefly summarized here, deal specifically with aspects of career decision making, training, and current professional activities as a consultant and include recommendations for improving various aspects of career development. Comparisons are drawn

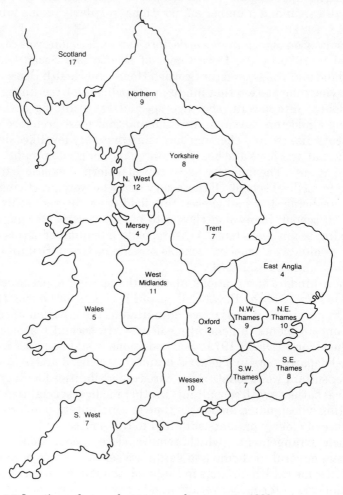

Figure 8-2 Locations of respondents to consultant survey, 1983.
Source: Barker, W. H., and Williamson, J. 1986. A survey of recently appointed consultants in geriatric medicine. *British Medical Journal* 293:896–99. Reprinted with permission.

between those appointed as full-time physician in geriatric medicine (PGM) and those appointed in the newer entity of general physician with responsibility for the elderly (GPRE).

A list of consultants appointed in the five-year period 1978–82 was compiled with the assistance of the regional health boards in England, Wales, and Scotland. An 80 percent response to the mailed survey questionnaire provided information on 130 consultants, 101 PGMs, and 29 GPREs. Respondents were well distributed throughout the land, roughly reflecting population distribution (see fig. 8-2). Median age at time of appointment was 35, and approximately 15 percent were women. A somewhat greater percent of GPREs graduated from medical schools in England and Wales (other than London), while greater percentages of PGMs qualified in Scotland or overseas.

Career Decision Making

Table 8-1 examines reasons for choosing a career in geriatric medicine. The most frequent response, offered by over 60 percent in both consultant subgroups, was "preference for working with a wide range of medical problems." Second and third most common were "good opportunities to obtain a hospital consultant post" and "positive experience in geriatrics during postgraduate training." These were followed in frequency by two answers dealing with the style of work: its multidisciplinary nature and its involvement with the community as well as the hospital. Smaller percentages of respondents selected family considerations, research and teaching opportunities, or a positive medical school exposure to geriatrics.

Table 8-1
Reasons for Choosing a Career in Geriatrics

	Total Responses (n = 130)	PGM (n = 101)	GPRE (n = 29)
Wide range of medical problems	67%	68%	62%
Consultant opportunities	46	50	41
Postgraduate experience	43	44	38
Multidisciplinary work	32	31	35
Societal needs	22	25	10
Hospital and community work	21	21	21
Family considerations	13	13	14
Research potential	9	8	10
Medical school exposure	5	5	7
Teaching opportunities	5	5	3

Source: Barker and Williamson 1986. Reprinted with permission.
Notes: PGM = physician in geriatric medicine; GPRE = general physician with responsibility for the elderly. Respondents were provided a list of the above answers and requested to select up to three most important in their career choice.

Geriatrics was reported as the first career preference by 49 percent of PGMs compared with 35 percent of GPREs, the majority of whom had initially preferred some other medical subspecialty. Respondents in both subgroups most frequently made a definite decision to pursue a career in geriatrics during the registrar and senior registrar stages of graduate training. A decision during medical school was mentioned only once. Over 50 percent of respondents indicated that their decision was strongly influenced by working with a specific individual who provided a positive role model in geriatric medicine.

Education and Training

Only 20 percent of respondents had received theoretical and 10 percent clinical education in geriatrics during medical school, most having graduated by the early 1970s, prior to the widespread incorporation of geriatrics as a standard part of medical school curriculum. Respondents averaged between five and six years total postgraduate training in general medicine and/or geriatrics before assuming their current posts. This training included an average of three years as senior house officer and registrar and two-and-a-half years as senior registrar. Participation in NHS management courses offered either at the University of Manchester or at the King's Fund College in London was reported by 70 percent. Training in geriatric medicine was rated as moderate or very good by 95 percent of respondents. Management and administration, various medical subspecialities, psychiatry in old age, and various aspects of rehabilitation were listed most frequently as areas in which further training would have been helpful.

Geriatrics Units

Geriatrics units in which respondents were working as consultants averaged 8–9 beds per 1,000 persons over 65 years of age, with an average of 2–3 beds per 1,000 located in district general hospitals and 4–5 beds per 1,000 in long-stay hospitals. Day hospitals, available in all but a few instances, averaged 1.3 places per 1,000 over age 65. All of these provisions, which differed on average very little between the two subgroups of consultants, were at levels approximating, but slightly below, the standards recommended by the British Geriatrics Society in 1982 (see Appendix B).

Over 80 percent of consultants in both subgroups reported having admission beds in district general hospitals. Important management elements found in almost all units included the existence of a central office for coordinating bed use, the conduct of regular multidisciplinary case conferences to review patient progress and care plans, and the use of a small percentage of the unit's beds for scheduled respite admissions of community-dwelling patients with heavy care needs. Median number of consultations on patients in their homes was five per week for both subgroups. On average, respondents reported spending less than one day a week in direct care of patients in long-stay beds. Regularly scheduled geriatric consultative liaison with general medicine was reported by 46 percent of PGMs and 69 percent of GPREs, with orthopedic surgery by 55 percent of PGMs and 41 percent of GPREs, and with psychiatry by 41 percent of PGMs and 17 percent of GPREs.

Table 8-2 lists ways in which consultants would change or improve their local geriatrics services. The most common suggestions include increasing acute beds and other facilities (including rehabilitation and long-stay beds and day hospitals), followed by increasing social services, rehabilitation therapists, and medical posts.

Academic and Administrative Activities

Table 8-3 summarizes selected teaching, research, and administrative activities. Roughly one-third of respondents in both subgroups reported regular involvement in medical student teaching, with one-half or more teaching house officers and one-fifth teaching general practitioners. Many reported involvement in one or more areas of research, with clinical research reported most commonly. Finally, one-half to two-thirds represented geriatric interests by serving on either hospital or community administrative committees.

A final open-ended question asked what reasons might be offered to medical students or house officers favoring a career in geriatric medicine. The answers, largely reflecting reasons the consultants

Table 8-2
Areas for Changing or Improving Geriatrics Services

	Total Responses (n = 130)	PGM (n = 101)	GPRE (n = 29)
Increase acute beds	27%	30%	17%
Increase other facilities	19	24	3
Increase social services	17	18	14
Increase rehabilitation therapists	15	16	14
Increase medical posts	15	17	10
Liaison with other departments	11	12	7
Psychogeriatric unit	8	10	3
Miscellaneous other	15	16	10
No response	8	4	24

Source: Barker and Williamson 1986. Reprinted with permission.
Notes: PGM = physician in geriatric medicine; GPRE = general physician with responsibility for the elderly. Respondents were given a list of the above answers, including "other," and requested to select up to three most important.

Table 8-3
Selected Teaching, Research, and Administrative Activities

	Total Responses (n = 130)	PGM (n = 101)	GPRE (n = 29)
Teaching			
Medical students	37%	38%	31%
House officers	48	45	62
General practitioners	20	22	14
Research projects			
Laboratory	19%	21%	14%
Clinical	66	71	45
Epidemiology	15	17	7
Health care	13	16	3
Committees			
Hospital	70%	70%	69%
Community	52	55	38
National	5	6	3

Source: Barker and Williamson 1986. Reprinted with permission.
Notes: PGM = physician in geriatric medicine; GPRE = general physician with responsibility for the elderly.

gave for their own selection of a career in geriatrics, included exposure to a wide variety of medical problems, good career prospects, a challenging career, and multidisciplinary and community involvement. Excellent opportunities for research was listed by 21 percent.

Comment

On the basis of this survey, recently appointed consultants in geriatric medicine or general medicine with responsibility for the elderly have received sound postgraduate training, approximating standards established by the Joint Committee on Higher Medical Training, and participate in a full array of medical services for the vulnerable elderly as called for in guidelines established by the DHSS in consultation with the British Geriatrics Society. Virtually all consultants surveyed routinely include domiciliary visits, multidisciplinary team case conferences, and scheduled respite admissions as strategies for meeting their patients' needs. Approximately half conduct regular consultative liaison services with departments of medicine and orthopedics and somewhat fewer with psychiatry. The majority of consultants have taken special courses dealing with organization and management of health and social services. Clearly the role of the consultant in geriatric medicine in Great Britain has evolved from its origins managing long-stay patients in chronic care institutions to a complex and dynamic practice of hospital and community medicine, much in keeping with the models proposed by various of its academic leaders (Williamson 1979; Pathy 1982).

Postgraduate training was generally rated well; nonetheless, a desire for further training in psychiatry, rehabilitation, and administration—three areas of particular importance in medical care of the elderly—was mentioned by a significant number. Each of these areas is specifically identified in recently stated JCHMT standards for senior registrar training programs in geriatric medicine. These needs are being addressed in part by the recent introduction of annual short courses on rehabilitation and psychiatry in old age, organized with BGS cosponsorship, by several departments of geriatric medicine.

Contrasting those appointed as full-time consultants in geriatric medicine with those appointed as general physicians with responsibility for the elderly, the major differences include a somewhat later time of career decision and smaller response to questions regarding improvements among the general physicians with responsibility for the elderly. Outweighing these differences are the striking similarities between the two groups of consultants with respect to the array of facilities and routine practices in their current consultant posts. This finding suggests that it is the special mix of medical and related needs of the elderly patient population, rather than one's job description, that prevails in determining the outcome of a choice of a career involving geriatric medicine.

While this survey, like the earlier study conducted by Hutt, Parsons, and Pearson (1981), finds that the decision to pursue a career in geriatrics occurs relatively late and usually not as a first preference, developments pertinent to more recent cohorts of medical students and trainees suggest significant improvements in recruitment to and enthusiasm for the specialty. These include nearly universal exposure of British medical students to formal education in geriatrics, with some evidence that this experience directly influences students toward choosing a career in geriatric medicine (Peach and Pathy 1982); the expanded number of opportunities for house officers to rotate on geriatric medicine units and work with geriatricians in district general hospitals; and the continuing decline in number of consultant opportunities in other medical and surgical specialities, relative to aspiring applicants (Lye 1982).

Surveys of physicians entering geriatric medicine training programs in the past several years have in fact found that an increasing percentage are graduates of British medical schools, that decisions to enter geriatric training are occurring at an earlier stage of career development, and that a majority prefer to practice full-time geriatric medicine as opposed to practicing general medicine with special

responsibility for the elderly (Brocklehurst 1984; Donaldson 1985).
Under the circumstances, one estimate suggests that the current rate
of entrants into geriatric training as senior registrars will yield
about the right number to fill the stated requirement of approximately eight hundred consultantships in Great Britain by 1990.

CHAPTER 9

The Development of Health Services for the Elderly in the United States to 1980

Medicare . . . provided a financing mechanism for individuals, a credit card for purchase of care, rather than any means for large-scale development in the organization of health services.
—R. STEVENS, 1971

The health and health-related problems of the elderly in the United States in the latter half of this century closely parallel those in Britain, yet as noted in chapter 1, the present organization of health services to deal with these problems is strikingly different in the two countries. In this chapter, the essential elements in the evolution of organized geriatrics services in Great Britain are briefly summarized, followed by a historical account of major developments in the United States to the beginning of the present decade, with discussion of the contrasting experiences of the two countries. In essence, where the British system melded acute and chronic care services for the elderly into one system, the United States pursued a course that accentuated the traditional schism between these two levels of care. Chapter 10 carries the story forward to the present and beyond by discussing a number of significant possibilities for the evolution of integrated, comprehensive health services for the elderly in the United States. Being experimental and innovative in nature, these developments do not reflect national policy. The final chapter commends these and related possibilities to the attention of U.S. policy makers and practitioners, with the thought that we might emulate the exemplary accomplishments of the British geriatric medicine movement.

The British Experience in Summary

From the time of its origins with the work of Dr. Marjory Warren and contemporaries, the overriding accomplishment of the geriatric medicine movement in Great Britain has been to remove the sharp lines of distinction between acute and chronic care and to foster a continuum of preventive, acute, rehabilitative, and continuing care services for the elderly. The movement began by bringing the dynamics of acute hospital medicine to public chronic care institutions, focusing upon thorough assessment, rehabilitation, and restoration of independence among chronically ill elderly persons who had been committed to a custodial existence in these institutions. With the coming of the National Health Service at midcentury, chronic care institutions were incorporated into a single hospital service alongside of the voluntary acute care hospitals, hence forging a direct link between emerging geriatric rehabilitation activities in the former and the mainstream of modern hospital medicine in the latter.

In response to national guidelines, hospital consultants in geriatric medicine, house staff, and multidisciplinary teams evolved to take responsibility for this sector of hospital care. Initially the role of geriatrics units was primarily to provide rehabilitation or chronic placement for disabled patients transferred from acute medical and surgical services. The past two decades have witnessed evolution of the practice of admitting elderly patients directly to designated geriatrics services in general hospitals on the premise that earlier comprehensive medical and functional assessment could prevent or reverse many disabling and costly consequences of aging and chronic disease. The fruits of these developments are evident from the variety of sites in which geriatrics services have been shown to reduce hospital admissions, lengths of stay, and bed blocking among elderly patients. The widespread adoption of rehabilitation-oriented day hospitals, scheduled respite admissions, house calls, and other progressive practices further reflect the innovative and energetic efforts of the leadership in the field of geriatric medicine. Geriatrics departments have also fully retained their fundamental roles in providing inpatient rehabilitation and continuing care for those elderly patients with such requirements.

While necessary and indispensible, the development of geriatric medicine units and specialists is not alone sufficient to explain the impact of the geriatrics movement. General practitioners have evolved a variety of health surveillance strategies targeted to vulnerable elderly members of their practices. Of fundamental importance also has been development of publicly funded community nursing and social support services that work in close liaison with hospital specialists and office-based practitioners to provide both acute and long-term care to elderly patients in the community.

The U.S. Experience to 1900

Directly mimicking the early British experience, beginning in the eighteenth century, American communities developed publicly funded poorhouses (almshouses) to provide shelter for lunatics, orphans, elderly, and other non-self-sufficient members of society. In the nineteenth century, specialized institutions evolved to meet the needs of various of these subgroups (insane asylums, orphanages, etc.), leaving growing numbers of aged and infirm persons to occupy the almshouses. In a number of cities the almshouses evolved into or were linked with public hospitals, in recognition of the heavy burden of chronic disease and disability among the elderly residents. These institutions included Philadelphia Hospital and Almshouse, later Philadelphia General Hospital; Long Island Almshouse and Hospital of Massachusetts; Bayview Asylum, later part of Baltimore City Hospitals; Monroe County Home and Infirmary, later Monroe Community Hospital; and Bellevue Hospital in New York (Carroll 1966; Freymann 1980, ch. 3). For those destitute elderly who primarily required shelter, there developed a network of public and charitable "old age homes" unaffiliated with hospitals (Haber 1983, ch. 5).

Concurrent with the evolution of almshouses, public chronic care hospitals, and old age homes, a voluntary hospital sector developed in the United States, again directly modeled on the British experience (see ch. 3). These hospitals were funded by the contributions of private individuals, as well as religious and ethnic groups, and were seen primarily as institutions for care and convalescence of persons suffering from accidents and short-term illnesses. Nonetheless, the needs of the old and chronically ill inevitably presented themselves to these hospitals.

The voluntary hospitals responded to the situation in several ways; many stipulated at the outset that their services were limited to those with curable conditions. Exemplary in this regard were the Pennsylvania Hospital, New York Hospital, and Charity Hospital in New Orleans. The latter declared in 1784 that it was for "persons who shall neither be incurable nor leprous" (Freymann 1980, 24). Other voluntary hospitals initially attempted to accommodate the frail elderly along with younger curable patients. Well-documented examples of these included St. Luke's Hospital in Chicago, Hartford Hospital (Connecticut), and the Roman Catholic Carney Hospital in Boston, which originally kept one of its five floors for "old people who may not be sick but come here for a home." However, by the turn of the twentieth century, these hospitals too excluded "incurable" old persons, as vividly exemplified in the decision by the Carney Hospital (Boston) that its function no longer included care for "chronic lingering inmates" (Haber 1983, 91). Voluntary hospitals had by this time become principally identified with the modern theories and practices of acute medicine, emphasizing new advances in bacteriology, immunology, and surgery. In absolving themselves of a role in chronic care of the aged, the voluntary hospitals emphasized that this role properly belonged to the emerging municipal and county old age homes. Not infrequently the hospitals took much of the initiative to encourage construction of such institutions, thus assuring themselves of the availability of custodial beds to which to transfer such chronic care aged patients as might initially present themselves to the acute hospital (Haber 1983, ch. 5). The popular American phenomenon of doctor-owned and -operated small proprietary hospitals, which proliferated in the nineteenth and early twentieth centuries, never became significantly involved with caring for the disabled elderly.

A distinct separation between institutional services for acute illness (generally involving the young) and long-term care (generally involving the aged) had thus developed by the beginning of the twentieth century. This configuration of service provision left unattended the needs of those elderly persons with chronic conditions for which neither the acute care hospital nor the long-term care institution was suited. To wit, what was missing, and continues to the present to be largely missing, was a continuum of services emphasizing rehabilitative and supportive care as well as acute and long-term care for elderly persons. At the beginning of the century, the need for such services bridging acute and long-term care was recognized but nonetheless not developed. Some leaders of medical progress in Boston and Baltimore were foremost among those who recognized the need.

The case in Boston is well captured in the following exerpts from a series of articles in the *Boston Medical and Surgical Journal* (forerunner of the *New England Journal of Medicine*) calling attention to the need for modern hospital services for elderly persons with chronic disease.

> It is time to enter a vigorous protest against the attitude of very many physicians, who are inclined to speak of the "old chronic" in terms almost of disparagement, and as an object unworthy of their serious consideration. . . . The great bulk of disease is chronic, and it is these chronic conditions which should peculiarly attract our attention as scientific physicians. Hence the perfectly natural tendency toward the establishment of hospitals for the incurable or slowly curable cases, which are usually refused admittance to our best municipal institutions. ("Hospitals for Chronic and Incurable Cases" 1896, 347)

> It should be evident to the most casual observer that disease, whether acute or chronic, demands the best service which modern methods can

give. It is hardly too much to say that the chronic sufferer often demands more care than the person ill with a self-limited disease. In the
second place, it is manifestly unjust that pauperism should be a necessary accompaniment of the misfortune of illness. It is one of the great
injustices of the present system that a poor man, hopelessly incapacitated, should be legally classified as a pauper. The hospital for chronic
disease should stand on precisely the same footing in this respect as the
hospital for acute disease. . . . Much as we need a hospital for the care
of advanced cases of tuberculosis, none the less essential is a hospital
for the care of all cases of chronic disease, absolutely irrespective of its
character. ("The Question of a Hospital for Chronic Disease" 1906, 445)

Such institutions were not to develop with any of the vigor with
which they were recommended in New England's mecca of medical
advances. In Baltimore the Quaker merchant John Hopkins, in a
letter expressing his thoughts on the future world-renowned medical
center that was to bear his name, called for inclusion of a progressive
care component:

Provide for a site and buildings . . . for the reception of convalescent
patients. You will be able in this way to hasten the recovery of the sick,
and to have always room in the main hospital building for other sick
persons requiring immediate medical or surgical treatment. (Quoted in
Freymann 1980, 53)

Initial plans for Johns Hopkins Hospital included one hundred
such convalescent beds to be connected to the main hospital. However, in the ensuing years this component was deleted from the plans in
favor of the exclusively acute care John Hopkins Hospital that
eventuated, the paradigm of the modern twentieth-century American medical center (Freymann 1980, ch. 3).

These various mechanisms whereby the elderly with chronic disease were, by the beginning of the twentieth century, segmented off
from the mainstream of progressive medical care are interpreted by
Haber (1983) as one manifestation of broad economic forces of industrialized societies which increasingly viewed aged persons as a group
with little productive role to play. In justifying their specific choice to
largely ignore the pursuit of the afflictions of chronic disease among
the elderly (and at the same time unwittingly to contribute to the
general societal tendency to separate the aged from the mainstream
of American life), the medical profession had, as elaborated by
Haber, formulated a nineteenth-century model of aging that supported such a stance: "Noting the changed anatomy, physiology, and
psychology of the old, doctors asserted that aging itself was a disease.
The elderly had little hope of returning to the physical or mental
state of the middle-aged" (p. 126).

From Social Security to Medicare

While the acute care hospital movement flourished during the opening decades of the twentieth century, little of consequence changed with respect to meeting the needs of the aged infirm until the 1930s. By 1920, approximately 0.5 percent of those over age 65, amounting to some fifty thousand persons, lived in old age homes, the institutional legacy of eighteenth- and nineteenth-century policies for dealing with society's unproductive and dependent members (Vladek 1980, ch. 3). For the rest there was little public or private provision against poverty and disability, save what they could provide for themselves. With the coming of the Great Depression, government officials realized that the archaic system and outdated philosophy of institutionalizing the destitute and chronically ill elderly was an untenable solution for the future. In the lead on this issue, the New York State Commission on Old Age Security in 1929–30 drafted a state law that became the model for the federal Social Security Act passed in 1935. In essence these new laws intentionally abandoned the traditional reliance on public institutions ("indoor relief") and made available instead direct cash payments with which individuals might secure food, shelter, and other essentials on their own. Supplemental grants for clearly destitute elderly persons were provided under the Old Age Assistance title of the Social Security Act ("outdoor relief"). The legislation specifically prohibited using these funds to support residents within public chronic care institutions. While thus inhibiting expansion of these institutions, the new law, with its focus upon providing adequate income for the majority of the elderly, made no explicit alternative provision for services to meet the special needs of disabled and dependent elderly persons. However, under the terms of the law, the supplemental Social Security funds could in fact be used to defray the cost of room and board in privately operated rest homes and boarding houses.

The Rise of the Nursing Home Industry

With the almshouse and its derivative public institutions receding from the American scene and modern hospitals disdaining to care for the chronically ill within their walls, proprietary nursing homes, under the stimulus of the Social Security Act, emerged to become the dominant solution to the needs of the infirm elderly. As aptly put by Freymann "with one stroke, completely without plan or intention," the nursing home industry as we know it today was born (Freymann 1980, 31).

In the 1950s, under pressure from the nonprofit and proprietary nursing homes, the Hospital Survey and Construction Act of 1946

(Hill-Burton law) and the Federal Housing Authority were broadened to provide advantageous financing for building or expanding public, nonprofit, and proprietary homes. Additional support came via the Medical Assistance to the Aged bill (Kerr-Mills) in 1960s and the Medicare and Medicaid legislation in 1965, all of which included some provisions to finance care in these various types of long-term care facilities. In response to these incentives, along with the original Old Age Assistance provisions of the Social Security Act, the nursing home sector mushroomed to some 20,000 facilities with over 1 million beds by the late 1960s. Proprietary homes, representing over 90 percent of the industry, grew in number from 1,200 facilities with 25,000 total beds in the late 1930s to over 19,000 facilities and 850,000 beds by 1967 (Freymann 1980, ch. 3).

Among the many unanticipated consequences of the massive growth of the nursing home industry were two of particular importance concerning the failure to develop an integrated continuum of health services for the infirm elderly. First was the absence of any functional linkage between these institutions and their aged infirm residents, on the one hand, and the acute hospitals and the medical profession on the other hand.* Second, given the strong bias toward expanding institutional long-term care for the elderly in the 1950s, 1960s, and 1970s, virtually no public policy was directed toward providing long-term support services in the community. Specifically, the development of public policy to support visiting nursing services in the United States in the first half of the century, while impressive, was largely limited to public health and crisis care of mothers and children in the home. There were no provisions for community support services comparable to home help services and the like that developed in Great Britain and other Western European countries (Mundinger 1983, chs. 3 and 4).

Thus in contrast to the British experience between the 1930s and 1960s when former Poor Law institutions became directly linked with general hospitals and related medical services, leading to the strong development of a continuum of services for the elderly, the major developments in the United States during this era saw the former public custodial care institutions largely replaced by a proliferation of private custodial facilities totally unaffiliated with the mainstream of medical care.

*There was, however, a technical linkage forged between the nursing home and hospital sectors as pointed out in the following statement from Vladek (1980, 45): "Inclusion of nursing homes into Hill-Burton—and thus into the jurisdiction of the Public Health Service, which administered the program—transformed them, by definition, into medical facilities. Nursing homes would never again be solely an extension of the welfare system; they now belonged to health policy as well."

Hospitals and Geriatric Rehabilitation

At midcentury a number of isolated efforts were made in the hospital sector, along the lines of those called for some fifty years earlier in Boston and Baltimore, and strikingly reminiscent of the initial development of progressive, rehabilitation-oriented geriatric hospital units in Great Britain. Interestingly, these efforts were premised on surveys that, like those of Marjory Warren and others in Britain, revealed large numbers of chronically institutionalized elderly for whom it was surmised that more vigorous rehabilitative and supportive services were in order. While, for lack of secure financing, few of these impressive projects survived beyond the demonstration period, their achievements serve as an important model of what needs to occur in this country.

A 1957 survey of some forty county hospitals in Michigan revealed large numbers of elderly patients with prolonged hospital stays for whom little more than custodial levels of care were being provided. A three-year research project was undertaken by faculty of the University of Michigan "to demonstrate and measure the extent to which dependency of aged patients in county hospitals could be reduced by rehabilitation of their functional abilities" (Rae, Smith, and Lenzer 1962, 463). A program consisting of assessment to identify rehabilitation potential, implementation of restorative services by physical and occupational therapists working closely with the nursing staff, and continuous supervision by an experienced physician was introduced in three of the hospitals. After one year, 34 percent of the study population had achieved significant functional improvements, compared with 5 percent of those in control hospitals; 20 percent of the former versus fewer than 5 percent of the latter had been discharged to home (Rae, Smith, and Lenzer 1962).

The renowned "continuing care" program undertaken by the Thayer Hospital, a progressive community hospital located in rural Maine, had somewhat similar origins and findings. Responding to a 1956 survey of unmet medical needs in Maine, which revealed a disproportionately large underserved population of elderly persons with chronic disabilities, the hospital established a Department of Continuing Care in the 1950s. Under the medical directorship of an internist interested in comprehensive medical care,* the department

*Interestingly, Dr. Harold Willard, the medical director, visited Great Britain in 1965 to compare his experience with progressive care for chronic illness with that of British leaders. His diary discloses lengthy discussions with several consultants in geriatric medicine, including Dr. Lionel Cosin in Oxford, in which the point is made that the problem is not chronic disease but "chronic neglect" of the elderly patient's needs by medical practitioners and educators (unpublished diary notes of H. W. kindly provided by Anne Willard, April 1985).

implemented a multidisciplinary program that provided assessment and demonstrably effective rehabilitation services to large numbers of elderly persons in the hospital, in nursing homes, and in their own homes. Commenting on the evident impact of the program, a reviewer in 1963 offered the prophetic observation, "while this work is in reality a pilot study for guidance of the State of Maine, it will be of service to other areas and eventually, *perhaps twenty-five years from now,* have wide application throughout the land, when 12 percent of our population will be over sixty-five years of age" (Willard and Kasl 1972, 131; italics added).

In Monroe County, New York, the combination of public concern for declining quality of care in the county chronic diseases hospital and a series of community surveys revealing many unmet chronic disease needs led to a community decision to forge a formal affiliation between the county facility and the University of Rochester School of Medicine in the early 1960s (Williams, Izzo, and Steel 1975). The expectation was that recruiting a vigorous research- and rehabilitation-oriented medical staff would solve many of the problems of the chronically ill and lead to discharge of some and avoidance of unnecessary admission of others. Through expansion that included an acute inpatient unit, the facility experienced considerable turnover in inpatients thanks to rehabilitation; reduction in admissions for long-term institutionalization was also achieved through an outpatient assessment and placement service (Williams et al. 1973). The institution continues to perform very successfully as a setting for chronic disease care and research, but as with other chronic care institutions (i.e., nursing homes), it remains administratively largely separate from the general hospital sector. And due to stringent terms of reimbursement, it has seen only limited development of rehabilitative care for the chronically ill.

Foremost among surveys was that conducted in several communities in the mid-1950s by the Commission on Chronic Illness, a voluntary organization created by the American Hospital Association, the American Medical Association, the American Public Health Association, and the American Public Welfare Association. Based on the survey's findings of extensive unmet needs among patients in nursing homes and public chronic care facilities, a national conference was held, with the following objectives:

1. Identify the requirements of the long-term patient in the various stages and severity of his illness.
2. Examine existing methods of providing care, explore new methods, and enunciate principles which should govern needed changes.

3. Suggest patterns for desirable relationships among services, facilities, and programs.
4. Recommend various ways to improve the financing of long-term care.
5. Establish direction and suggest next steps for local, state, and national programs for the care of the long-term patient. (Commission on Chronic Illness, 1956, xii)

Recommendations at the end of the commission's voluminous report entitled "Care of the Long-Term Patient" addressed most of the issues essential in defining and addressing chronic illness in a progressive manner. Central to the recommendations was the need to integrate the care of the chronically ill into general medical services, with particular emphasis on rehabilitation. Toward these ends, significant reforms and developments of community care, general hospital services, and education of health professionals were called for. (Selected text from these recommendations is reproduced in Appendix H.)

Perhaps the most prodigious effort to achieve the commission's recommendations was a project sponsored by the American Hospital Association and described in a monograph entitled "A Chronic Disease Unit in a General Hospital: Analysis of Six Years' Operating Experience" (Littauer, Steinberg, and Gee 1963). This project was based at the Jewish Hospital of St. Louis, a five hundred–bed voluntary teaching hospital that became affiliated with a local chronic care institution for the express purpose of improving provision of medical services to the residents of the latter institution. Due to lack of on-site diagnostic services, medical staffing, and so forth, the chronic care facility was closed and its patients transferred to a sixty-three-bed "chronic medicine" unit established within the general hospital. Through this arrangement, vigorous medical and rehabilitative care, including physical and occupational therapy, were provided to this formerly neglected population of elderly, chronically ill persons. Over a period of years, beginning in 1951, the average length of stay was reduced from over 600 days, with 80 percent of discharges due to death, to average stays of 140 days, with 31 percent of discharges due to death. A list of the wide range of chronic diseases among patients treated on this service is shown in table 9-1. The unit was unable to continue beyond the period of special project subsidy because the unit's services were not covered by Blue Cross and other private third-party payors or by public Old Age Assistance grants.

From the well-documented success of this project, the author, an internist with a strong interest in chronic disease and rehabilitation medicine, drew several conclusions remarkably similar to those that

Table 9-1
Distribution of Diagnoses of Patients Discharged from a Division of Chronic
Medicine, 1957–1962

Diagnostic Category	Total	1957	1958	1959	1960	1961	1962
Total	911	125	138	121	159	168	200
General cerebral							
arteriosclerosis	100	13	19	7	19	20	22
Congestive heart failure	52	11	7	7	10	8	9
Coronary insufficiency	68	7	17	13	12	9	10
Cerebrovascular accident	149	29	22	20	17	18	43
Parkinsonism	31	4	4	2	5	5	11
Multiple sclerosis	12	3	3	1	2	1	2
Neoplasms	227	32	41	30	42	42	40
Arthritis	21	2	2	2	2	7	6
Pulmonary disease	14	3	0	0	3	4	4
Renal disease	14	2	1	3	3	3	2
Fractures (hip)	98	4	9	23	22	18	22
Amputations	36	6	6	4	7	6	7
All others	89	9	7	9	15	27	22

Source: Adapted from Littauer, Steinberg, and Gee 1963. Reprinted with permission.
Notes: Patients are recorded under only one diagnostic category. In cases where diagnoses were multiple, the condition that contributed most to the need for care in the chronic disease unit is the one recorded.

emerged from the analogous experiences of Dr. Warren and others in Great Britain. These included:

Long-term care services properly belong in the professional and administrative purview of the general hospital. Chronically ill patients require access to the same medical, nursing and technical staffs, and to the same facilities and equipment, as do short-term "acute" patients. . . .

Because of superior resources of personnel, equipment, and physical plant, the services rendered to chronic-disease patients tend to be more comprehensive and of higher quality when incorporated in the organic envelope of the general hospital than when provided by an independent chronic disease institution.

While a chronic disease unit is considered one gradation of care in the over-all general hospital complex, it also has implications for care at the community level. Homes for the aged, nursing homes, home care programs, and social agencies should be made aware of this resource as one more definitive level in the spectrum of patient-care facilities. It is essential that close working relationships be developed with all these institutions and agencies operating in the field of long-term care. . . .

This analysis of the operation of a long-term medical service in the framework of a voluntary general hospital has pointed up the need for additional or complementary services. For example, the practice of geri-

atrics as a medical specialty should be recognized, since it is important
to identify this form of practice as an organizational entity. (Littauer,
Steinberg, and Gee 1963, 52, 54–55, 57; italics added)

Medicare and Medicaid: The First Decade

The historic passage of Title 18 (Medicare) and Title 19 (Medicaid) of
the Social Security Act in 1965 represented a major and unprecedented commitment on the part of the federal government to provide
comprehensive health care for an entire sector of the population, the
elderly. Contained within this legislation were, superficially speaking, most of the essential elements of a continuum of services—
physician services, acute and convalescent hospital care, home care,
and long-term institutional care. Conspicuously lacking from the
legislation, however, was any mechanism to facilitate effective integration of these elements into one system.

Described by Marmor as the product of incrementalist policy making or the "politics of legislative possibility," the Medicare and Medicaid legislation reflected on the one hand a recognition of the real and
undisputed need of the chronically ill elderly and their families for
financial relief from the burden of costly health services. On the
other and more fundamental hand, the legislation reflected an accommodation of the existing physician, hospital, health insurance,
and nursing home establishments by primarily providing vastly expanded financing to support prevailing patterns of health service
delivery (Marmor 1970). An examination of policies with respect to
specific service components reveals the built-in obstacles that
thwarted development of a continuum of care appropriate to needs of
the aged with chronic disease.

Hospitals

Universal coverage for acute hospital care for the elderly to be financed through the established payroll-tax social insurance mechanism of Social Security was the principal focus of the Medicare
legislation (Medicare Part A). Hospitals were to be reimbursed from
the Medicare Trust Fund on a cost basis much like existing practices
under Blue Cross and commercial health insurance plans, with existing third-party payors (primarily Blue Cross) employed to serve as
fiscal intermediaries for the government.

An innovative and potentially very constructive Medicare initiative that went beyond traditional hospital third-party coverage
was the concept of the extended care facility (ECF). Broadly defined
on the basis of experiences such as those reviewed in the previous
section ("Hospitals and Geriatric Rehabilitation") and statements

from the American Hospital Association,* an ECF consisted of a unit within an acute general hospital, or in a nursing home formally affiliated with a hospital, to which patients might be transferred for a period of postacute convalescent care before discharge. While conceptually very similar to the linkage of acute and rehabilitative inpatient services that evolved in British geriatrics units, the motivating force behind the ECF provision of the Medicare legislation was in fact not so much to provide appropriate rehabilitative and restorative services as to reduce the lengths of stay of convalescing elderly patients in costly acute care beds. This became apparent within the first two years of the legislation's implementation when, faced with unexpectedly high utilization and costs of acute as well as extended care hospital benefits, the Social Security Administration introduced a number of stringent criteria for a patient to qualify for ECF reimbursement. These ultimately appeared in the form of a nine-page document issued by the Social Security Administration in 1969 (Intermediary Letter 371), which provided fiscal intermediaries with detailed guidelines for classifying a given patient's care needs as "covered" or "noncovered" under the ECF provision. Coverage was restricted to those patients receiving high-intensity skilled medical-nursing or physical rehabilitation services; others requiring lower-intensity rehabilitative care, as was commonly the case with hospitalized elderly persons, were placed in the newly defined category of "custodial care,"† not coverable by Medicare (Archer 1970). The impact of such regulatory measures is succinctly captured in the following comment from David Stewart of the Rochester (New York) Blue Cross, a Medicare fiscal intermediary: "From any point of view, E.C.F. benefits simply do not exist in the form everyone originally contemplated. The guidelines make it very clear that in order to get benefits, patients in E.C.F.s have to be receiving care very nearly on the level with acute care in hospitals. Few such patients ever go to E.C.F." (Thurlow 1972, 187).

In measuring the impact among some twenty-two Medicare-certified ECF units in the state of Pennsylvania, Archer (1970) documented a 47 percent decline in Medicare-reimbursed ECF days fol-

---

*"Community hospitals must become even more comprehensive or 'general,' extending the range and depth of their services to include . . . effective rehabilitation programs. In most cases, the need for . . . chronic illness units and long-term care nursing units is great; and we believe these are best provided either directly under the auspices of, or in close affiliation with, a general hospital" (American Hospital Association 1962, 1).

†Medicare prohibits payment for "custodial care," defined in the *Medicare Handbook* as follows: "Care is considered custodial when it is primarily for the purpose of meeting personal needs and could be provided by persons without professional skills or training; for example, help in walking, getting in and out of bed, bathing, dressing, eating, and taking medicine."

lowing the 1969 directive. Nationally there was a decline in Medicare reimbursement for ECF care from over 1 million billings totaling $348 million to fewer than 400,000 billings totaling $156 million. To summarize from Vladek's treatise: "From the time of Intermediary Letter 371 on, Medicare was no longer a significant factor in the nursing home industry. At great cost, with great confusion, and not inconsiderable pain to thousands of old people and their families, Medicare was finally doing relative to nursing homes, what its sponsors had first intended—hardly anything" (1980, 57).

Physicians

The second leg of the three-legged stool of the Medicare and Medicaid legislation was the provision for coverage of physician services (Medicare Part B). With politic adherence to the principle of noninterference with prevailing medical practice, the law provided for reimbursement of physician services on the basis of "customary, prevailing and reasonable charges," with existing health insurance organizations again serving as fiscal intermediaries.

One distinctly new role the legislation conferred upon physicians was that of serving as certifying authorities for services provided to the elderly at virtually all levels of care. Accordingly, physician orders and approval became the basis not only for reimbursible hospital and medical office services, but for certifying home care and nursing home services. The criteria for physician certification were, in the case of home care services, narrowly medical and therapeutic in nature, and in the case of nursing home care, bureaucratic and hierarchical in nature.

Specifically lacking from the Medicare law were any incentives for physicians to make visits to frail elderly patients in their homes. Nor did the legislation encourage or facilitate physicians to work as part of a multidisciplinary team with other professionals in meeting the broad medical and social care needs commonly experienced by the elderly, in the home, hospital, and nursing home setting. None of these low-technology activities was sufficiently remunerative when working under a fee-for-service system, which primarily rewards discrete items of service and procedures.

Home Care

As in the case of the ECF provision, the Medicare legislation, in both Parts A and B, included ostensibly progressive provisions for home care services. However, as developed in depth by Mundinger (1983) in a book entitled *Home Care Controversy: Too Little, Too Late, Too Costly,* these provisions were narrowly defined to apply only to skilled care needs that derived directly from an acute hospitalizing or potentially hospitalizing illness. Under Medicare A, such services were to be provided following discharge from hospital in hopes of expediting discharge and cutting overall costs to the Medicare program. Under Medicare B, home health services were to be provided in lieu of hospital admission. In both instances the services had to be ordered by a physician and certified as medically necessary in the treatment or convalescence of short-term acute illness. Furthermore, services had to include the involvement of one or more skilled professionals from the fields of nursing, physical therapy, and speech therapy.

Missing from the home care program was any coverage for long-term health maintenance or social support in the home for chronically disabled elderly persons. This lack was made explicit in the *Medicare Manual,* which states under home care: "The aged person who is feeble and insecure (without a medical condition causing it) doesn't qualify" (Mundinger 1983, 41).

This narrowly medical focus of the Medicare home care benefit, which was strongly supported by physicians and hospitals, with no significant consultation with the nursing or social work professions, has had a number of untoward consequences. First, according to Mundinger's study (1983, ch. 4), it led to a proliferation of proprietary home care organizations prepared to market relatively costly and profitable skilled care services. These in turn displaced many voluntary visiting nursing organizations that had during the preceding decades become increasingly engaged in providing low-cost long-term health and social support to homebound elderly.

The second and ultimately most costly consequence of the limited scope of home care benefits for the elderly under Medicare was the failure to develop an infrastructure of community-based health maintenance and social support services as viable alternatives to nursing home placement. This folly would be recognized in the following decade when both the massive growth in the nursing home bed supply and cost and the increasing problem of "backup" of chronic care elderly patients in acute hospitals at great cost to Medicare gave rise to a spate of efforts to develop community-based "alternative" long-term care services (see ch. 10). Finally, having conferred upon physicians the responsibility for initiating and supervising home care plans for Medicare recipients, the legislation made no provision for reimbursing physicians for such time-consuming functions. This lack of remuneration has contributed to physicians' tendency to play their role in home care in a perfunctory manner, ratifying plans developed by others rather than becoming actively interested and involved in such services (Koren 1986).

This experience with home health care developments in the United States contrasts sharply with policy initiatives in Great Brit-

ain at approximately the same time. There, existing community
nursing services were encouraged to integrate with general practitioners to better coordinate care for intercurrent medical problems
with ongoing health monitoring of chronically ill elderly persons
living in the community (see ch. 7).

Nursing Homes

With the exception of the limited coverage of extended care facilities
under Medicare, as discussed earlier, longer-term nursing home care,
like its home care counterpart, was explicitly excluded from Medicare, the "universal health insurance program for the elderly." Nursing home care was, however, included as one of the mandated services
to be provided under the third major component of the 1965 Social
Security Amendments, Medicaid.

Medicaid itself received relatively little attention in the debate
preceding enactment in 1965. In essence the Medicaid program represented a successful effort on the part of its principal author, Congressman Wilbur Mills, to consolidate under one program a variety of
existing federal-state grant-in-aid programs to finance medical and
medically related services for the indigent. Encompassed within its
scope was the 1960 Kerr-Mills Medical Assistance to the Aged program and in turn the long legacy of treating public provision of
institutional care for the chronically ill elderly as a means-tested
welfare service. The inclusion of nursing home coverage in the Medicaid bill, with little debate or consideration of future consequences,
has been described by Vladek as the "sleeper" in the 1965 Social
Security legislation.

While serving to keep the nursing home sector distinctly separate
from the mainstream medical sector, inclusion in the Medicaid program did lead to considerable structural reform within nursing
homes per se. This reform largely took the form of setting and implementing standards, a process approached vigorously by the Senate
Special Committee on Aging and with varying degrees of rigor by
federal and state government offices responsible for nursing home
affairs (Vladek 1980, ch. 3). Standard-setting efforts were particularly directed to building codes, safety and environmental hygiene
considerations, staffing patterns, and reimbursement rates. With
these came increasingly tough regulations, including periodic accreditation review under a set of long-term care facility guidelines
developed by the Joint Commission on Hospital Accreditation. Little
attention was given to service roles to be played by the medical profession, other than to impose a set of perfunctory requirements that
each facility have a medical director and each resident have a physician of record who must visit on a regular basis to review and author-

ize care plans and medications. A regrettable consequence of these standards has been the tendency to define nursing home operations on an inappropriate medically oriented model in which the physician, who is infrequently present, is cast in the role of central decision maker and supervisor of the work of others who are present full time. Such an arrangement stands in stark contrast to the multidisciplinary medical-social model developed in British geriatrics services (see chs. 4 and 5) which has been repeatedly recommended by critics of U.S. nursing home care (Kayser-Jones 1981; Johnson and Grant 1985, ch. 10).

The Impact of Medicare and Medicaid

The major measurable impact of the Medicare and Medicaid legislation was a massive and rapid rate of growth in public expenditures on health. This was apparent within the first year of the legislation's enactment and continued thereafter as annual rates of increase ranged between 10–20 percent. These expenditures were reflected in very significant increases in rates of hospitalization, admission to nursing homes, and visits to physicians' offices among the elderly, as well as expansion of hospital and nursing home facilities, and growth in the size and composition of the health personnel sector (Gornick et al. 1985).

Despite the essentially fiscal character of the legislation in removing financial barriers to customary medical and institutional services, it was reasonable to postulate that such a large infusion of money might lead to improvement in the overall organization and quality, as well as the quantity, of health care provided to the elderly. A wide variety of formal studies as well as informal observations during the first ten to fifteen years following the legislation afford useful, if unsettling, insight into this postulate.

Among the earliest and most comprehensive assessments was a series of surveys of all aspects of the health delivery system in metropolitan Kansas City. The findings, compiled at intervals of two and six years after implementation of the Medicare and Medicaid laws, consistently revealed little evidence of constructive change in the delivery system. In summary, most physicians had not altered methods of practice, though they were aware of certain inadequately met needs of elderly patients; hospital administrators reported few Medicare-related modifications of their services other than some limited trials with ECF units; nursing home beds increased appreciably, but there was no significant effort to coordinate care between nursing homes and hospitals; home health services increased initially, but the number of Medicare-reimbursed services actually declined over time due to increasingly restrictive reimbursement regulations. Finally, the local Comprehensive Health Planning Agency, created under the 1966 health planning amendment to the Public Health Services Act for the express purpose of coordinating the various public and private components of the health care system, was found to have had no discernible impact in fulfilling its stated purpose insofar as a system of care for the elderly was concerned (Coe, Brehm and Peterson 1974).

The functioning of various components of the overall delivery system has been the subject of many other studies. Foremost among these were numerous surveys assessing the match between elderly persons with chronic or long-term-care needs and the availability of services appropriate to these needs. This strategy, pioneered by Berg and others (1970) in Monroe County, New York, in the early 1960s, consistently found, both before and after the 1965 legislation, large percentages of such patients receiving inadequate or inappropriate care. Most impressive among a series of such studies reviewed by Dunlop (1976) was the finding that between one-fifth and one-third of residents of skilled- and intermediate-care nursing homes were receiving inappropriately high levels of care. In the vast majority of instances it was concluded that such persons could be supported in the community if formal long-term home health services were available.

Other surveys suggested that as many as 2.5 million noninstitutionalized elderly individuals were in need of varying degrees of continuing home care. In fact, as of the early 1970s, fewer than 10 percent of this population were actually receiving such services, according to a survey conducted by the Social Security Administration. It was surmized that the tendency to overutilize high-level institutional long-term care and underutilize home care services was primarily the result of the restrictive institutionally and medically biased reimbursement policies of Medicare and Medicaid (Dunlop 1976).

This phenomenon was further manifested in the acute hospital sector in the form of the "administratively necessary" stay (also referred to as "backup" or "alternate care" status). These terms referred to those hospitalized patients, usually elderly, who, following an acute care episode reimbursible under Medicare, could not be discharged due to the lack of posthospital home support services or nursing home placement. The dearth of the former and the frequent difficulty in finding available nursing home beds often left such patients languishing in acute care beds for months.

The dominant and distorting nature of reimbursement policies was apparent even among elderly persons who received home health care. In a revealing study, Mundinger (1983) carefully chronicled

Medicare-reimbursed "skilled" nursing care provided to a series of fifty patients by one home health agency in the northeast United States. Unreported, and hence unknown to the Medicare fiscal intermediary, over half of the patients did not meet the strict Medicare criteria for home health care, and virtually all received some services explicitly excluded from Medicare coverage. In this instance, and doubtless in many others, professional decision making by visiting nurses overrode regulatory restrictions in the interest of providing services appropriate to the patients' needs.

Finally, a number of observations shed light on the provision of medical care to nursing home residents. In most respects, the evidence revealed a pattern of indifferent and often marginal quality of physician services. Various studies showed high rates of drug misuse, particularly the employment of psychotropic agents to control behavior, unattended infections, unevaluated incontinence, and other broad areas of medical neglect among nursing home patients (Pastore et al. 1968; Rango 1982). Generally this neglect was attributed to physician disinclination and lack of financial incentive to provide care in the nursing home setting that equaled the same high standards applicable in the office or hospital setting. A further impressive phenomenon reflective of this outlook was the very high rate at which nursing home patients were transferred to acute hospitals: approximately 250 hospitalizations per 1,000 beds per year, based on National Nursing Home Survey data (U.S. Dept. of Health, Education, and Welfare, National Center for Health Statistics 1979). This rate contrasted with a rate of 50 or fewer hospital transfers per 1,000 beds per year from the continuing care institutions under geriatric coverage in Britain (ch. 6).

In 1975 the Senate Special Committee on Aging, Subcommittee on Long-Term Care, published a document entitled "Doctors in Nursing Homes: The Shunned Responsibility," which attributed medical neglect of patients in nursing homes to both the lack of interest and training in care of old and chronically ill patients and the relatively poor reimbursement for providing such services. That such neglect was not a necessary and inevitable state of affairs was demonstrated in a number of instances, both academic and nonacademic, in which high-quality medical care was provided by salaried physicians working in long-term care settings. Such experiences, which often included teaching and research activities along with excellent medical care, have been described (Ingman, Lawson, and Carboni 1978; Rodstein 1979; Libow 1982; Williams 1981).

Comment

One of the most telling assessments of the condition of health services for the elderly in the United States in the Medicare-Medicaid
era, and particularly suited to the theme of this book, was provided
by Dr. Lionel Cosin (1971), a leader of the British geriatrics movement, in testifying before the Senate Special Committee on Aging in
1971. Invited to advise the legislators in their quest for solutions to
the costly and controversial "American System of Long-Term Care,"
Cosin was quick to point out that the problem posed by nursing homes
could not be effectively understood and attacked without taking into
account the whole spectrum of services for the infirm elderly, as was
done in Great Britain. Asked to elaborate on this point, Dr. Cosin
provided a detailed description of the operations of the geriatric medicine services he directed in Oxford, England, which bore a striking
resemblance to the hospital-based, community-linked continuum of
services originally proposed in the BMA's 1947 report, "The Care and
Treatment of the Elderly and Infirm" (see ch. 3).

Of the American situation, and the nursing home dilemma in
particular, which he had observed in travels to many parts of the
United States, Cosin drew the following contrast with the British
approach:

> There is no planning. The whole thing is amorphous. Someone wants to
> build a 100-bed nursing home. All they need is 100 patients. But you
> can always get 100 neglected patients who haven't been properly as-
> sessed medically, psychologically and socially, treated by the appropri-
> ate means of rehabilitation, resettled into the appropriate community
> situation, not in a nursing home, and given a continuing program of
> care and responsibility. . . . What are we doing when we bring one
> patient up to the day hospital? Affecting a wide system—treating a
> patient—but also affecting a wide system of intercommunication.
> What are we doing when we say, "Well, we'll take grandma in for 2
> weeks so you can have a vacation?" There is a great deal of interchange
> of thought going on. . . . This is the point, you see. Here the whole thing
> is episodic. Seven days and you're out. Out where? Well, it doesn't really
> matter as long as they're out. Because there is no continuing clinical or
> sociomedical responsibility. This is the basic difference. (P. 1395)

The following comments by Dr. Cosin, respecting the role of the
hospital, the physician, the family, and community, all bespeak a
keen observer's recognition of the need for more appropriate and
better-organized services in this country:

> There are many pessimistic views concerning the hospital treatment of
> the elderly which stem from poor organization, both past and present,

in this branch of sociomedical work. *It fails primarily to provide facilities for rehabilitation of the elderly.* Interesting research problems on available pathological material are no doubt important. However, the first concern must be to provide the maximum benefit to each and every inpatient, regardless of age, in the minimum of time. There is little point in organizing purely medical units for the solution of sociomedical problems. . . . We've got to come down to the responsibility of the physician, in planning patient care on a short term and a long term basis. . . . I do not think necessarily the fault is the fault of the family or the community. It's in large part the fault of the organization and the provision of the care. (P. 1396; italics added)

When asked toward the end of the hearing, "What would you say would be the main problem with the American system of elderly care?" Cosin was brief but emphatic:
"Too much money resulting in neglect."

CHAPTER 10

The 1980s
Toward Comprehensive Services in the United States?

By the beginning of the 1980s, the dilemma of "too much money resulting in neglect," as portrayed in Dr. Cosin's testimony of a decade earlier, had been greatly magnified in the United States health sector in general, and in services for the elderly in particular. National expenditures on health care had increased from $75 billion representing 7.5 percent of the Gross National Product in 1970 to over $250 billion representing over 9 percent of the GNP in 1980. A major portion of the increase was attributable to hospital and nursing home services for the elderly, largely funded by Medicare and Medicaid, respectively. In the face of a national economy increasingly troubled by inflation, recession, and a growing national debt, the element of neglect could no longer persist. Accordingly, state and federal government, as well as the private sector, embarked on an era of tough legislation, regulation, and other measures intended to stay the rising expenditures in the health sector. This has been accompanied by a prevailing conservative mood favoring a decreased role of government and increased role of the private corporate sector in providing health services (Starr 1982).

Running concurrent with the economic and political forces driving the cost-containment movement have been a series of innovative proposals for financing and organizing health services for the elderly. While these have invariably been cognizant of the need to be cost conscious, they represent in a more fundamental sense some real efforts to rethink and restructure services to more appropriately meet the full spectrum of health care needs of the infirm elderly.

Policy Proposals

Policy recommendations proposed from several perspectives at the beginning of the decade bear testimony to the growing quest for organizational reforms in the acute and chronic care services for the elderly. It is significant that many of these (along with countless other recommendations for change in recent years) are directed to "long-term care." Clearly the area of greatest neglect has been the continuing care of the chronically disabled elderly persons, which for lack of any coherent policy has been relegated to nursing homes and like custodial institutions.

A seminal article entitled "Long-Term Care for the Elderly and Disabled: A New Health Priority," by Anne Somers (1982), a widely respected health policy analyst, begins with the following observations:

> Of all the difficult health-care issues facing the nation today, none is more complex or urgent than the formulation of a viable policy of long-term care for the elderly and the chronically ill and disabled. The tragic irony of the existing neglect is clearly evident in the plight of millions of frail and dependent elders, rejected by both Medicare and Medicaid as well as by most private carriers of health insurance, even as the costs of these programs soar. . . . Although many of the current remedial proposals recognize the importance of long-term care, they appear to be prepared to settle for a second-class program, *separate in both organization and financing from the mainstream of acute care.* (P. 221; italics added.)

Citing the many built-in obstacles to continuity of care in a divided system, as discussed in chapter 9, the article proposed extending the Medicare program as follows: "The need for continuity between acute and long-term care should be explicitly recognized, and a defined schedule of benefits for long-term care—both institutional and home-based—should be included. Medicare (rather than Medicaid) reimbursement for such services would be provided" (pp. 223–24). Among the elements of this proposed solution, three essentials stand out: payment of providers would be on the basis of fixed prospectively negotiated rates, long-term care services in home or institution would be coordinated by community agencies responsible for assessment and continuing cost-effective case management, and the patient's primary physician would have major responsibility for managing both acute and chronic phases of care.

In a proposal that comes directly from the medical profession, the American College of Physicians' (ACP) Health and Public Policy Subcommittee on Aging (1984) issued a position paper entitled "Long-Term Care of the Elderly." Its opening statements, defining the scope of the issue, are strikingly reminiscent of the definition of geriatric medicine promulgated by the British Geriatrics Society some years

earlier and endorsed by the Royal College of Physicians (1977), the
British counterpart of the ACP:

> Long-term care refers to the medical and support services needed to
> attain an optimal level of physical, social, and psychological function-
> ing by persons who are frail and dependent due to chronic physical or
> mental impairments. It includes services to prevent avoidable deterio-
> ration of health, to treat acute exacerbations of chronic illness, to
> maintain the greatest possible independence, and to restore the person
> to the optimal level of functioning that can be sustained. Long-term
> care is often mistakenly seen as only nursing home care or home
> health care. It, nevertheless, includes diagnostic, preventive, re-
> habilitative, supportive, and maintenance services in both institu-
> tional and noninstitutional settings. (P. 760)

Again, as in Somers' proposal, the lack of an organized continuum
of services is identified as the critical problem to be solved:

> At present, there is not a comprehensive system of long-term care for
> the elderly in the United States. A confusing, fragmented, and expen-
> sive system exists that contains both gaps and duplication of services.
> Consequently, many elderly do not receive the services they need,
> while others receive services inappropriately. . . . Reimbursement pro-
> cedures, both public and private, tacitly recognize the existence of two
> separate systems of health care: one for acute care and another for
> long-term care. Such a division is unrealistic and results often in inad-
> equate responses to the medical needs of the elderly. (P. 760–61)

Proposed reforms under an integrated system of care, while not
addressing financing mechanisms, include many of the elements of
the continuum of services found in Britain:

> A full array of services should be available through an integrated long-
> term care system that enables the family (or surrogates) to meet the
> changing, but continuing, needs of the elderly in the least restrictive
> settings possible. These supportive services should include in-home
> assistance, such as provision of hot meals, visiting nurse services, and
> homemaker services; community services, such as senior citizen cen-
> ters, community meals, and geriatric day rehabilitation hospitals; and
> institutional services, including a variety of housing arrangements,
> intermediate care facilities, skilled nursing home facilities, acute care
> hospitals, and mental health facilities. Such a continuum of care would
> better ensure that the elderly obtain appropriate services. . . . The re-
> imbursement system should foster, not impede, networking among
> hospitals and nursing homes. (P. 761)

An enlightened, progressive view of the physician's role is espoused, much in keeping with roles evolved by geriatricians and general practitioners caring for the elderly in Britain, and sharply contrasting with the prevailing narrowly defined medical role in long-term care in the United States described in chapter 9:

> The internist, family physician, and general practitioner should continue to be the principal providers of medical care for the elderly. Long-term care, however, often requires a range of services that extend beyond the usual scope of traditional medical and nursing care. Personal care is usually required for activities of daily living (eating, dressing, bathing, toileting). Other required services include housing, social and recreational activities, physical therapy, and mental health care. Dental, vision, hearing, and podiatric services are also necessary. To provide these services most effectively, a team involving professionals in multiple fields may be needed. . . . The team approach requires leadership, but not autocratic direction. Most daily caring for the frail elderly is provided by nonphysicians and it makes sense for all team participants to apply their professional expertise without undue burdensome requirements for physician approval. (P. 763)*

A policy proposal prepared by a team of physicians and health economists, the Harvard Medicare Project, and published in 1986 encompasses most of the service elements contained in the Somers and ACP proposals and in turn addresses the critical issue of financing such a system of comprehensive health care for the elderly. In essence the Harvard proposal calls for expanding the Medicare program to encompass chronic care services, with financing to be derived primarily from a combination of funds from a proposed 1 percent addition to Social Security taxes on employers and employees and shifting to the Medicare program federal general revenue funds currently used to pay for nursing home care in the Medicaid program. This carefully developed proposal, in accomplishing its fundamental goal of creating a single comprehensive system of health care for the elderly, emphasizes three important related goals: containment of expenditures; fairness to elderly persons, health care providers, and others affected by the program; and simplification of administration by removing many arbitrary barriers between sources of coverage for various services.

*A complementary position paper from the ACP (1986) Health and Public Policy Aging Subcommittee on "Home Health Care" reviews evidence of the shortcomings in provision of home care services in the United States and makes a series of very progressive recommendations for improving availability, financing, and physician involvement in this specific component of health services for the elderly.

Several further policy proposals, while acknowledging the need for a fully integrated continuum of services for all elderly persons, have focused principally upon the select subset of disabled elderly who require permanent long-term supportive care. These proposals have been developed by persons primarily concerned with sponsoring or managing various community-based alternatives to nursing homes, who recognize that effective reform calls for more than simply shifting some nursing home services to the community.

Foremost among these is former U.S. congressman Barber Conable, who, in his position as senior Republican member of the House Committee on Aging, introduced the Medicare Long-Term Care Act on several occasions prior to retiring in 1984. The proposed bill, which was never enacted, called for an amendment to the Medicare program whereby persons paying an additional premium (as is the case of the Medicare B provision for physician services) would be entitled to a variety of home-based social support services and/or institutional care, along with usual medical services, at such time as they might become sufficiently disabled to require such services. The essential objective of this policy proposal in overcoming the Medicare program's narrow medical criteria for coverage was its commitment to "provide protection against the costs of long-term care, both institutional and noninstitutional, without concern about drawing an arbitrary and unnecessary line between health care services and nonhealth care services." The key organizational reform consisted of the creation of community-based "long-term care centers" to act as both coordinating and paying agencies for all required services (Conable 1982).

A variation on the Conable bill was advanced by several persons involved in government-sponsored efforts at cost containment in the long-term care area. In an article entitled "Management and Financing of Long-Term-Care Services: A New Approach to a Chronic Problem," Ruchlin, Morris, and Eggert (1982) proposed the creation of local-area management organizations (LAMOs) to coordinate the planning, delivery, and payment of the full array of medical, rehabilitative, and custodial maintenance services required by persons with certifiable functional deficits and long-term care service needs. The LAMO would pool for the target population all existing public funds earmarked for acute and long-term care (Medicare, Medicaid, other) and serve in a case management capacity, emphasizing less costly home-based services over institutional services whenever possible.

While policy proposals such as those offered by Somers, the American College of Physicians, and the Harvard Medicare Project on the one hand, and those contained in the Conable and LAMO initiatives, on the other hand, differ in their target populations, they have in common the objective of unifying the delivery of acute and chronic care services. Other recently promulgated approaches to reforming health services for the elderly would maintain the financing and provision of acute and long-term care as two separate programs and seek to build incentives for greater efficiency and more sound financing for each. Such proposals have been developed from the perspective of both the Medicaid and Medicare programs.

In the case of Medicaid, a National Study Group on State Medicaid Strategies, faced with the fact that expenditures for nursing home care of the elderly were eroding funds meant also to finance health services for the nonelderly poor, produced a position paper entitled "Restructuring Medicaid: An Agenda for Change" (1983). Concluding from its deliberations that the Medicaid program had grown in ways that were never anticipated and that there was "no conceptual, practical or political justification for maintaining the current combination of acute health care and long-term care services in one program" (p. 3), the study group recommended that the program be restructured into two separate systems of care: a federally financed program to provide uniform basic health and medical care benefits for all low-income individuals and a state-administered system for providing long-term care services. From the perspective of the beleagured Medicaid program, such restructuring would allow more rational program planning and financing. From the perspective of health service policy for the infirm elderly, this proposal would only reinforce the long-standing inappropriate separation of chronic care from the continuum of acute and rehabilitative care. This point was briefly stated in a critical letter to the *New York Times,* dated 22 February 1984, entitled "Missing 'Linchpin' in a Medicaid Proposal," in which the contrasting experience in Great Britain was cited (see figure 10-1).

In 1985 Dr. Otis Bowen, the newly appointed secretary of the Department of Health and Human Services, proposed a two-phase strategy for protection of Medicare recipients against catastrophic costs of acute and long-term care, respectively. The first phase, to be funded through an additional Medicare Part B premium, was designed to assure funding for the relatively rare but financially catastrophic situation in which an individual's inpatient and outpatient costs exceed the prevailing upper limits of acute and skilled care coverage under the current Medicare program.* Under the second phase, individuals would have the option during their productive years to contribute to a new Social Security fund called an individual

*See Appendix I for delineation of Medicare-covered benefits.

Missing 'Linchpin' in a Medicaid Proposal

To the Editor:

The recommendations of the National Study Group on State Medicaid Strategies, reported in The Times Feb. 5, would perpetuate and aggravate the inappropriate division of medical services for the elderly between "acute" and "long-term" care that currently prevails in the country.

Missing from this simplistic, fiscally motivated "blueprint for action" is an appreciation for rehabilitation, a critical dimension in medical care of many elderly persons. (Fortuitously, an excellent article on rehabilitation medicine appeared in the magazine section of the same issue of The Times.)

Rehabilitation medicine, which involves physical and occupational therapy as well as psychological and social support for patients in the postacute, convalescing stage of illness, enhances patients' chances that they will be able to remain in their own homes rather than having to go to a nursing home. Active incorporation of "geriatric rehabilitation" into the continuum between acute and long-term care has for decades served as the linchpin of medical care of the frail elderly in Great Britain, where far more such persons are able to return home after hospitalization.

Before proceeding to deliver to Congress a plan that changes nothing but the mechanism for funding our current limited and fragmented medical services for the elderly, the study group should give some hard thought to developing a continuum of acute, rehabilitation and long-term care.

WILLIAM H. BARKER, M.D.
Rochester, Feb. 6, 1984

The writer is an associate professor in the University of Rochester's Department of Preventive, Family and Rehabilitation Medicine.

Figure 10-1 Letter to the New York Times, 22 February 1984. Reprinted with permission.

medical account (IMA), comparable to a tax-deferred individual retirement account (IRA), which would provide insurance against catastrophically high long-term care expenses later in life. Quick to point out that "it is strictly a fiscal proposal," and one with considerable appeal from the point of view of both state and federal government for whom the consequences would be "cost neutral" and possibly cost saving, the authors concluded with what can only be an indicting statement from the perspective developed in this book: "It is bold in that it provides a form of comprehensive health insurance *without disturbing existing delivery systems*" (Bowen and Burke 1985, 45; italics added).

A number of initiatives to develop private long-term care insurance have appeared in recent years. While varying in extent of cost sharing and duration of coverage, all are premised upon contributing to an insurance fund during one's productive years to assure the availability of financial protection specifically against potentially prolonged, costly care for chronic illness late in life (Meiners 1983). Private long-term care insurance would relieve taxpayers and consumers of many of the costly and offensive features associated with Medicaid-funded long-term care. It would also help to redress the cruel disillusionment experienced by the many elderly who mistakenly assume that Medicare provides coverage for long-term nursing home needs.* There are nonetheless significant barriers to such developments (Davis and Rowland 1986, ch. 4). Included among these are a variety of untested marketing and financial risks to the insurance industry. Most important is the tendency, for reasons of fiscal control, for long-term care insurance plans to focus primarily on nursing home benefits and very little on long-term care services in the home, which would generally have greater appeal to elderly persons. Again, as in the two previously discussed government-initiated proposals, this private initiative would perpetuate the existing inappropriate institutionally based and segregated approach to chronic care of the elderly.

Service Innovations

All of the foregoing reflect the growing thoughts of policy makers and health care providers toward developing more comprehensive, appropriate, and fiscally sound approaches to providing acute and chronic care services for the elderly in the country. Despite the considerable effort expended on such thinking, no concerted policy-making efforts in this direction appear to be in progress at this time.† However, the past few years have witnessed numerous public and private sector initiatives toward developing and evaluating innovative health service delivery modalities, the fruits of which may be incorporated into some future national comprehensive health care policy. Broadly speaking, these initiatives may be considered at two levels. First are those that have been largely developed from the perspective of one or more particular sectors in the spectrum of services for the elderly, including hospital, nursing home, community care, medical personnel. Second are those organizational initiatives to develop model comprehensive health care delivery systems that link fiscally and functionally the full spectrum of acute and chronic care services, for example, the social health maintenance organization (SHMO). A selective review of these health service innovations reveals a number of promising opportunities for the United States to

---

*A national survey conducted in 1983 under the auspices of the American Association of Retired Persons (1984) revealed that 79% of elderly persons surveyed believed incorrectly that Medicare would pay for all or a substantial part of an extended stay in a nursing home.

†Several current initiatives to develop legislation for a comprehensive health program in the United States and the possibility for these to garner significant political support are discussed at the end of ch. 11.

attain an organized continuum of appropriate services for its elderly, in some ways comparable to what has successfully evolved in Great Britain.

Hospitals

As the best-funded, most sophisticated, and prominent health service modality in our society, hospitals have always been heavily used by the elderly and their physicians, with particularly dramatic increases since passage of the Medicare legislation. Representing 11–12 percent of the population, those over 65 years of age account for some 40 percent of hospital days, with 25–30 hospitalizations per 100 persons per year and a substantial number involving persons with multiple readmissions (Lubitz and Deacon 1982; Anderson and Steinberg 1984). Typically, hospitalizations for elderly persons have averaged two to three days longer than for persons under age 65. Furthermore, substantial numbers of these costly hospital days are accounted for by patients who, no longer qualifying for Medicare-reimbursed care, are placed on alternate care or "backup" status, awaiting nursing home placement. It has been estimated that patients awaiting nursing home placement occupy as many as 5–10 percent of acute hospital beds in the country at any given time (U.S. Dept. of Health and Human Services, Office of the Inspector General 1980).

Confronted with seemingly insatiable growth in hospital expenditures, in the early 1980s the government increased cost sharing by Medicare beneficiaries and in 1983 enacted the well-known Prospective Payment System for reimbursing hospitals under Medicare. Paying a predetermined fixed price for each hospital admission according to its Diagnosis Related Group (DRG), this system puts a premium on shortening hospital lengths of stay. Hospitals have simultaneously faced pressure from the increasing number of prepaid health plans, which by their nature seek to avoid hospital admission and keep lengths of stay to a minimum.

The collective effects of these developments have induced the hospital sector to take vigorous steps toward developing new service modalities. According to surveys conducted by the American Hospital Association in 1981 (Evashwick, Rundall, and Goldiamond 1985) and again in 1985 (personal communication, William Reed, January 1987), the majority of hospitals in the country have recently introduced some form of special services for elderly patients. In brief, these services consist of various ways in which hospitals have sought to anticipate special rehabilitative and posthospital support needs of elderly patients. While on the one hand such services may simply serve to expedite discharge in the interest of protecting the hospital financially, on the other hand, under the best of circumstances, patient functional levels and posthospital care may be enhanced. Three particularly interesting areas of innovation to be considered in this context are inpatient geriatric evaluation and rehabilitation programs, hospital–nursing home affiliations, and hospital sponsorship of community-oriented case management services.

Taking the cue from the British experience, a number of approaches to implementing inpatient geriatric evaluation and rehabilitation services have been undertaken recently in general hospitals in the United States. Premised on the concept of screening acutely hospitalized elderly patients to identify those most likely to benefit from rehabilitative as well as acute care, such specialized geriatric services have been incorporated into the acute hospital in the three different ways shown in figure 10-2.

The simplest and least obtrusive approach, signified by C on the figure, has been introduction of geriatric consultation services. These services, modeled on successful experiences in Edinburgh and elsewhere in Great Britain (see chs. 4 and 6), involve consultation by a

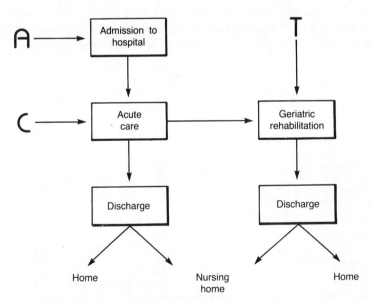

Figure 10-2 Potential intervention by special geriatrics services in the course of acute hospital admission in the United States.
A = Admit to acute geriatrics service
C = Geriatric Consultation on acute medical and surgical services.
T = Post-acute transfer to special geriatric rehabilitation unit.

multidisciplinary team (e.g., physician, nurse, social worker, others with expertise in geriatrics), preferably early in the hospital stay, to assess the patient's potential for rehabilitation, assist with planning for posthospital placement, and advise on management of certain medical and medically related problems. A community-wide project in Monroe County, New York, in which geriatric consultation teams were introduced in six general hospitals, was associated with a 21 percent decline in the census of disabled elderly patients "backed up" on alternate care status in acute hospital beds and awaiting posthospital placement. Table 10-1 summarizes the ten most frequent recommendations offered among the 366 patients referred in the course of this project. These recommendations graphically depict the spectrum of largely nonbiomedical needs that frequently play an important role in determining the outcome of care of the elderly patient in hospital. On followup it was found that 50–70 percent of recommendations were successfully acted upon. In a number of instances, failure to carry out recommendations was attributable to inadequacies of the health care system (Barker et al. 1985).

Descriptions of implementation of geriatric consultation services in several other acute hospital settings have reported similar experiences leading to improvement in patient functioning and posthospital placement (Steel and Hays 1981; Campion, Jette, and Berkman 1983; Lichtenstein and Winograd 1984). One of these studies, however, reported the disappointing finding that there was no difference in rate of hospital readmission between consult patients and

Table 10-1

The Ten Most Frequent Geriatric Team Recommendations among 366 Patient Consultations in a Monroe County, New York, Project, 1982

Recommendations	Percent of Consults[a] (n = 366)	Percent Carried Out[b] (n = 182)
Care plan change	49	53
Medication change	30	51
Home care referral	29	48
Physical therapy referral	27	55
Skilled nursing facility referral	16	47
Patient/family education	16	67
Socialization	15	69
Bowel/bladder training	13	64
Subspecialty referral	11	55
Rehabilitation facility referral	11	58

Source: Barker et al. 1985. Reprinted with permission.

[a] Average of three recommendations per consultation.

[b] Based on 182 cases in which medical record documentation was sufficient to permit a determination.

a control group during a one-year follow-up period. A likely basis for this failing of acute inpatient consultation is succinctly presented in the authors' discussion, "It appears that, to be effective, interventions must be more longitudinal and more community-based. Such control over after-care is cited as a key to the success of British geriatric consultation services" (Campion, Jette, and Berkman 1983, 795).

The modality labeled T on figure 10-1 consists of a special hospital-based or affiliated unit to which patients are transferred for geriatric rehabilitation following acute care on a medical or surgical service. This unit represents a contemporary reincarnation of an entity originally envisioned by medical leaders in Baltimore, Boston, and elsewhere late in the nineteenth century and intermittently introduced under special funding in various sites in the United States in the 1950s and again briefly in the form of Medicare-inspired extended care facilities in the 1960s—all reviewed in chapter 9. Such units have recently been established or given renewed vigor in a variety of hospital settings, including Veterans Administration hospitals, academic medical centers, chronic disease and rehabilitation hospitals, and rural community hospitals (Applegate et al. 1983; Lefton, Bonstelle, and Frengley 1983; Shaughnessy and Tynan 1985; Liem, Chernoff, and Carter 1986).

The Geriatric Evaluation Unit (GEU) at the Sepulveda Veterans Administration Medical Center in Los Angeles is perhaps the best known and most carefully evaluated of these. This fifteen-bed unit is operated by a full-time medical, nursing, and social work team, with part-time participation by physical and occupational therapists, a clinical psychologist, dietician, community health nurse, and others on the medical center staff. Approximately 10 percent of elderly hospitalized patients are referred to the unit, following screening for geriatric rehabilitation potential. In a series of studies from a randomized clinical trial, Rubenstein and colleagues (1984, 1985) have reported the following findings:

1. GEU patients experienced significantly lower mortality (24 percent versus 48 percent), likelihood of nursing home admission (27 percent versus 47 percent), and fewer overall acute hospital or nursing home days over a one-year follow-up, significantly greater improvement in functional status and morale, and lower average cost of care, in comparison with control patients.
2. GEU patients with greatest measurable benefit from the program were those over age 75, those with poorest functional rating at admission, and those with heart disease.

3. Aspects of GEU care that independently contributed to survival included using specific rehabilitation services and making new medical diagnoses.

An interesting variation on the "transfer" model is illustrated by a twenty-bed rehabilitation-oriented long-term care program at the University of Rochester Medical Center in which primary care nurses, working under a medical director, have major responsibility for implementing rehabilitation for postacute elderly patients with skilled-nursing-home level-of-care needs. Averaging forty- to fifty-day stays, the majority of several hundred patients admitted to this unit have shown significant improvement in physical and/or mental function and been discharged either to home or to a low-dependency long-term care institution. One major problem involving about 20 percent of the unit's patients has been the development of acute medical episodes necessitating backtransfer to an acute hospital service (personal communication, Anthony Izzo, March 1986). This experience, while verifying the potential role for nurses in implementing a geriatric rehabilitation unit, also points out the importance of active medical participation in this phase of care (as is routinely the case in British geriatrics units), hopefully to reduce the necessity for transferring patients back and forth between acute and rehabilitation units.

The third modality for incorporating inpatient geriatric rehabilitation into the acute hospital, labeled A on figure 10-1, consists of designating all or part of an acute medical admitting service as an acute geriatric unit. This approach has the advantage of locating disabled acutely ill elderly patients in a rehabilitation-oriented environment from the outset of hospital admission and is in keeping with current advances in acute hospital geriatric care in Great Britain as described elsewhere in this book. To date, relatively few such undertakings have been reported in the United States. Among these experiences, two based in nonacademic community hospitals have reported interesting findings from controlled evaluations. In the first of these demonstrations, ten-bed acute "geriatric special care units" were established in two hospitals in the suburbs of Boston, under funding from a private foundation. Each unit was staffed by a multidisciplinary team, using the primary nursing model, and was available to all physicians with attending privileges at the hospitals. It was postulated that, in comparison with a control group of patients admitted to the traditional acute medical service, those ill elderly patients admitted directly to the rehabilitation-oriented acute units would have shorter, less costly hospital stays, would lose fewer of their activity of daily living skills during hospitalization, and would be less likely to be admitted to nursing homes or be rehospitalized following discharge. Preliminary analyses suggest some significant reduction in overall cost and average lengths of stay among patients on the special units (Collard, Bachman, and Beatrice 1985). The second demonstration involved a similar 12-bed unit developed within the acute medical services of a 194-bed community hospital in Rochester, New York, and evaluated with support from the Rochester Area Hospital Corporation. Evaluation of the experiences of the first 120 admissions compared with those of control subjects admitted to the usual acute medical service revealed statistically significant improvement in functional status, particularly ambulation, and a lower average cost of hospitalization. While length of stay was not effected, the lower average cost was primarily accounted for by less intensive use of laboratory testing and ancilliary services among patients admitted to the acute geriatrics program (Boyer, Chuang, and Gipner 1986).

From these several demonstration experiences, geriatric evaluation and rehabilitation services implemented in U.S. acute care hospitals appear to be both effective and efficient in their impact upon patient functional status and health service utilization (Rubenstein, Rhee, and Kane 1982), and as such emulate this aspect of British geriatrics services. Importantly, however, virtually all of these programs have required Medicare waivers or special subsidy from short-term grants or other sources outside of existing reimbursement mechanisms. (The Veterans Administration hospital services represent an exception in this regard, as discussed subsequently.) Lacking the status of a designated medical specialty that might be reimbursed on a fee basis, and involving very significant participation by nonphysician health professionals who are not paid on a fee-for-service basis, a hospital-based geriatrics service must largely be reimbursed from existing hospital revenues.

To further frustrate the prospects for dissemination of the demonstrated successes of hospital-based geriatric rehabilitation services, the regulations governing hospital payments by DRG category under the Medicare Prospective Payment System specifically limit special waivers for rehabilitation to six medical conditions (amputation, arthritis, head trauma, hip fracture, spinal cord injury, and stroke). These diagnoses fail to account for the majority of hospitalized elderly who may benefit from hospital-based geriatric evaluation and rehabilitation units. When petitioned on this point by concerned physicians with evidence to support their case, the Health Care Financing Administration (HCFA) rejected the appeal with the unsubstantiated statement, "we believe that, in most cases, inpatients treated in geriatric assessment and rehabilitation units would have at least one of the listed conditions" (U.S. Dept. of Health and Human Services, HCFA 1984; personal communication, Drs. Leo Cooney and Richard Lindsay, November 1985).

In an era of tightening expenditures for hospital care, it is clear that hospitals and third-party payors will have to be committed to providing appropriate financial support if special geriatrics services are to play a serious role within their walls. It further must be recognized, as pointed out in an earlier instance, that special geriatrics services restricted primarily to hospital inpatient activities will generally have only limited longer-term impact in maintaining patient functional status and assuring optimal posthospital care. This once again begs the issue of establishing functional linkages between the acute and long-term care sectors. Hospital initiatives in this regard are discussed as they relate to the broader set of issues currently addressed through innovative developments in the nursing home and community care sectors.

Nursing Homes

The well-chronicled rapid and costly rise of nursing homes to become the dominant source of formal long-term care in the United States has, for reasons alluded to in chapter 9, been accompanied by significant gaps in the quality of medical and related care provided to the residents (Vladek 1980; Johnson and Grant 1985). The problem of high and increasing expenditure on nursing homes has been approached by a number of strategies, ranging from state regulations to prevent the increase in number of nursing home beds to the undertaking of numerous federal- and state-sponsored demonstration projects seeking cost-effective community-based alternatives. The latter are discussed subsequently in the section "Community Care." To date none of the various measures directed at cost containment has emerged as a clear and acceptable answer to this most vexing problem (Lave 1985).

In terms of gaps in quality of care for nursing home residents, two significant medically related deficiencies have begun to receive some long overdue innovative attention. The first of these is the paucity of appropriate on-site medical care for handling intercurrent acute and subacute illness episodes. Second is the relative dearth of geriatric rehabilitation practices, despite the fact that rehabilitation has long been one of the purported roles of nursing homes (Institute of Medicine 1986, Appendix B).

The most conspicuous, costly, and potentially preventable component of acute medical care for nursing home residents is the frequent transfer of patients to acute hospitals. The national annual rate of approximately 250 such hospitalizations per 1,000 nursing home beds translates into some 400,000 hospitalizations per year (U.S. Dept. of Health, Education, and Welfare, National Center for Health Statistics 1979). Many of these hospitalizations result from acute episodes, particularly infections, that might have been prevented or treated within the nursing home (Brown and Thompson 1979; Van-Buren et al. 1982; Irvine, VanBuren, and Crossley 1984). A significant number also involve patients whose underlying advanced degree of disability might, on ethical and medical grounds, mitigate against heroic acute medical intervention at time of a life-threatening intercurrent illness (Levenson et al. 1981; Hilfiker 1983; Wolff et al. 1985).

Potentially avoidable hospitalization has repeatedly been associated with a lack of active medical attention to the care of acute illness within the nursing home setting. That low levels of transfer to hospital from long-term care settings may be satisfactorily achieved by linking these settings with geriatric medicine services bears out this point (see chs. 5 and 6). Several innovative approaches to improving medical involvement in care of acute illness in the nursing home in the United States have in fact been shown to reduce the rate of hospitalization. These include a physician–nurse practitioner partnership that contracts to provide continuous medical care to a large number of nursing home residents (Master et al. 1980); an academically affiliated nursing home that provides coverage for residents by primary care teams of medical residents and nurse practitioners under supervision of a geriatrican (Wieland et al. 1986); a hospital-based medical group that has adopted and evaluated the impact of individualized care planning for a panel of nursing home patients (Mott and Barker 1987); and a Medicare waiver project that provides special financial incentives to nursing home staff and attending physicians to treat acutely ill residents within the nursing home in lieu of transfer to hospital (Zimmer et al. 1987). The latter study estimated significant cost savings to Medicare without apparent untoward outcome from the patient's perspective.

In addition to innovative approaches to avoiding unnecessary hospitalization, progressive nursing homes are increasingly introducing institutional policies for preventing or managing various predictable and commonly encountered medical problems. These include programs to deal with urinary incontinence, falling, influenza vaccination, diabetes monitoring, and others.

Though availability of rehabilitation services is one of the standards required for nursing home accreditation, and in principle rehabilitation in nursing homes is coverable under Medicare and Medicaid, the record reveals that this service is infrequently provided. At a national conference on the teaching nursing home, it was noted that fewer than one-third of all skilled nursing facilities in the country provide any type of rehabilitative care (Brody 1985). This lack may be attributed to two phenomena. First, the field of rehabilitation medicine has developed as a medical specialty primarily identified with acute hospitals and specialized rehabilitation hospitals. While a few of these programs have focused on the special rehabilitation needs of the disabled elderly, the field has primarly served a younger population of disabled persons, with a view to vocational as well as physical rehabilitation (Gritzer and Arluke 1985; Brody 1986). Under these circumstances, relatively few medical or nonmedical rehabilitation professionals (e.g., physical, occupational, and speech therapists) have been involved in the nursing home setting.

The second major barrier to rehabilitation services in nursing homes has been the variable and generally restrictive coverage by Medicare and Medicaid for rehabilitation in skilled nursing facilities. In essence this is a variation on the hospital extended care facility experience of the late 1960s (see ch. 9). The inhibiting effect of such reimbursement policies on development of rehabilitation services for nursing home patients has been thoroughly documented by Feder and Scanlon (1982). Despite these barriers, the recent implementation of the Diagnosis Related Group (DRG) based system for hospital reimbursement and the proposed analogous case mix reimbursement system for nursing home care pose interesting possibilities for developing rehabilitation services in nursing homes. Under the pressure of the DRG system to discharge patients as quickly as possible, acute hospitals are inclining toward establishing formal affiliations with nursing homes. This would provide a lower-cost setting to which to transfer elderly patients who are in need of further inpatient convalescence prior to returning home. To assure that such nursing home–based convalescent beds do not become blocked, there will be incentives to provide rehabilitation services to elderly patients in these settings (American Health Care Association 1986). Under a long-term care case mix reimbursement formula, based on resource utilization groups (RUGS), currently under trial in several parts of the country, nursing homes would receive differential rates according to intensity of care required by their residents. Patients requiring and receiving daily rehabilitation services involving licensed rehabilitation therapists would command relatively high reimbursement rates, commensurate with the higher expense of providing such services (Fries and Cooney 1983).

While these consequences of reimbursement reform may bring greater attention to rehabilitation in the nursing home sector, it is likely that this development will apply only to a relatively small proportion of the elderly who, while admitted to nursing homes, are ultimately destined to be discharged home. For the large proportion of elderly nursing home residents who are destined to remain institutionalized, some encouraging rehabilitation initiatives independent of reimbursement pressures have emerged recently. Of particular note among these has been development and successful testing of the so-called responsive care-giving model, which is premised upon active involvement of lower-level attendant staff in providing basic rehabilitative care to the residents with whom they work most closely. The following concluding statement from a project report, commissioned by the Institute of Medicine, speaks well for the potential contribution of such services:

> Conducting the development and evaluation of a rehabilitation focused technology of nursing home organization and management in six predominately Medicaid funded nursing homes has convinced us that existing standards of care can be substantially upgraded throughout the nursing home industry, with no additional expense to providers and payors. Our research clearly shows that nearly all nursing home residents are capable of much greater functional independence than their caregivers either realize or foster, and socially significant reversals of functional dependencies among even "bedfast" and chronically impaired residents occur in just days to weeks, when their lower level nurse aide attendants are organized, trained, and supervised to routinely provide rehabilitative services in the context of their usual caregiving interactions. (Ward 1984, 33)

Clearly this important work, based upon sensitive observation and pursuit of alternative outcomes for the institutionalized elderly, echoes the early work of Warren and others, which has been central to the modern geriatrics movement in Great Britain (see ch. 3). Stimulated by the experience of this project, the National Association of Health Care Facilities, representing some nine hundred publicly owned nursing homes in this country, has launched a major quality-of-care initiative to encourage widespread implementation of such fundamental rehabilitation services (personal communication, Benjamin Latt, July 1985). A related undertaking has recently been proposed by the American College of Health Care Administrators, the national professional society for long-term care administrators (personal communication, Kathleen Griffin, ACHCA, 21 January 1987).

Community Care

Development of community-based services for the elderly in the United States has commanded a great deal of attention in the past decade. This attention has primarily resulted from efforts by the

Medicare and Medicaid programs to find cost-saving alternatives to
the heavy use of hospitals and nursing homes by chronically ill elderly. Despite the considerable attention given to these efforts on the
part of federal and state government and some private foundations,
little consensus has been reached and few substantive changes in the
structure of the delivery system have resulted.

Two essentially different strategies have guided the development
and evaluation of community-based services (fig. 10-3). The first,
primarily representing the perspective of Medicare, focuses upon
expediting discharge of frail elderly patients from the acute hospital
by providing short-term skilled nursing care at home. This long-
standing concern has been intensified with the implementation of
the DRG-based Prospective Payment System of hospital reimbursement and the increased involvement of prepaid plans in providing
care for the elderly in the past several years. The second strategy,
representing primarily the Medicaid perspective, focuses upon avoiding admission of long-term care patients to nursing homes. This area
of activity has been the most vigorous for the past decade, ever since
policy makers were awakened to the unanticipated growth in Medicaid-funded nursing home use that occurred in the early 1970s.

Evaluations of innovative community care programs have yielded
highly variable results. Some appear to have succeeded as less costly
alternatives to hospital and nursing home care, while many have not.
Some have reported improvement in patient functioning and/or reduced morbidity or mortality, but many have not (Zawadski 1983;
Vogel and Palmer 1985). Underlying these mixed findings are a variety of study design problems peculiar to health services evaluation,
much of which does not lend itself to true experimental design
(Hughes 1985). This situation is particularly aggravated by the complex mix of social, medical, and mental health problems commonly

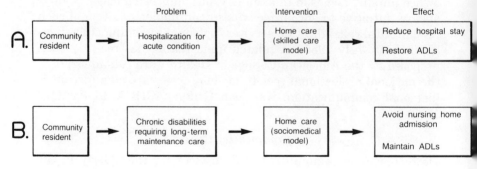

Figure 10-3 Two models for delivering and evaluating community-based services for
the elderly.

found among the elderly persons whom the programs are designed to serve. Given that such multiple dimensions may influence outcomes, programs that primarily focus on social support but lack a medical component, or vice versa, may fail to achieve their intended result.

In the absence of definitive evidence of cost saving or other expected outcomes, it is nonetheless important to recognize that the quest for noninstitutional alternatives has introduced to the United States health care delivery system a number of important new modalities for consideration in meeting the needs of its elderly. This becomes apparent in a selective review of these efforts.

Community-based long-term care alternatives for the elderly originated in special legislative provisions from the 1960s and 1970s. Specifically, the Older Americans Act passed in 1965 provided limited funds for a variety of homemaker, transportation, day care, and other social support services to be provided to any community-dwelling elders in need of such, and to be administered by state or regional agencies on aging. Title 20 of the Social Security Act, passed in 1974, authorized a similar range of social support services; however, only those elderly persons with demonstrated low-income status (e.g., receiving Supplemental Security Income) were eligible. Both of these programs have remained relatively small, have existed as social services largely independent of the Medicaid and Medicare programs, and have received little evaluative study (Rich and Baum 1984). Recognizing the potential for these types of services to impact favorably on physical and functional health and in turn to reduce use of hospital and/or nursing home services, in the mid-1970s the Medicare program initiated a multicenter randomized trial to assess benefits of homemaker and/or day care services offered to community-dwelling Medicare enrollees who were in need of continuing care. Results over a one-year period showed significantly better physical functioning, contentment, and mortality experience among certain subgroups of the study population; however, in the aggregate there was no measurable decrease in use of nursing home or hospital, and in fact the overall average health and health-related costs were higher for the experimental groups (Wan, Weissert, and Liveratos 1980; Weissert et al. 1980). From this and other experiences it was concluded that the support services were serving more of an additive than substitutive role and that in the future such projects should be more carefully targeted to those in the community at highest risk of using costly institutional services (Weissert 1985).

Subsequently, a series of further Medicare- and Medicaid-sponsored community care alternative projects has been undertaken. The first wave of these included the Monroe County (New York) Long-Term Care Program (ACCESS), the Connecticut Triage Program,

Project OPEN in San Francisco, the Georgia Alternate Health Service Project, and several others that have been well described and analyzed (Zawadski 1983; Vogel and Palmer 1985). In essence, these projects all represent variations on the emerging notion that enrollees in community care alternative programs should be certified by prior assessment to have disability levels that would qualify for nursing home admission. This assessment modality has since become a mainstay of most community long-term care programs. Case managers or case management agencies assume responsibility for first determining a person's eligibility and need for long-term support services and then serve as the brokering agent, organizing, reimbursing, and monitoring the various home care and other services deemed necessary to maintain the individual in the community. A further iteration of this modality was embodied in the Medicaid-sponsored Channeling Projects in which several organizational variations of case management were tested among projects in some ten different locations around the country. As noted earlier, evaluations of these collective efforts have failed to yield convincing evidence of success in terms of improved health or reduced health care expenditures. What does appear favorably affected are client sense of contentment and well-being and the level of stress experienced by family and other involved caretakers (personal communication, William Weissert, March 1986). These "softer," less quantifiable parameters have not, however, been adequately measured.

A final currently active Medicaid-sponsored initiative to generate and evaluate community care alternatives, known as the Home and Community-Based Care Program, consists of a provision under section 2176 of the federal government's 1981 Omnibus Budget Reconciliation Act, which authorizes state governments to substitute various community care modalities for institutional long-term care under the Medicaid program. This highly flexible provision now embodied in the Medicaid authorizing legislation has been adopted to varying degrees by virtually all states in the country. The service modalities being developed and used under this authorization include the following, in order of greatest frequency of use: case management, homemakers, adult day care, respite care, personal care, structural modification to home environment, and home health aides (Lave 1985). In contrast to past approaches, deployment of community home care and day care services paid for by Medicaid under this new program do not require physician authorization.

In summarizing and reflecting upon the cumulative experience with community-based alternatives over the past decade, the several salient conclusions to emerge include:

1. The need to target such programs to those at highest risk of long-term institutionalization.

2. The need to measure impact of programs in terms of client satisfaction and care giver well-being as well as the more quantifiable measures of mortality, morbidity, disability, service utilization, and cost.

3. The need for flexibility in deciding which services are coverable, whether they be social or medical, and where they are to be provided.

4. The need for a gatekeeper–case management entity to orchestrate case finding, assessment of client need, care planning and coordination, and ongoing monitoring to assure the dual objectives of providing both an efficient and appropriate mix of services.

Acute care hospitals, situated at the center of the health care system and beset with the challenges of an increasingly aged constituency, as reviewed earlier, have inevitably become involved in planning and operating community-based support services for the elderly. The potentials and essential imperative for such involvement are captured in several brief remarks from participants in a symposium entitled The Distinctive Role of the Hospital in the Continuum of Care for the Elderly, presented at the thirteenth International Congress of Gerontology in New York City in July 1985:

Hospital or community are not alternatives but complement each other. (J. Williamson)

The hospital has a natural role in geriatric care. It is a natural entry point into long-term care. (R. L. Kane)

The hospital not only houses a unique technological capacity but also possesses a unique capacity to mobilize and coordinate diverse professional, technical, and managerial resources. (B. Vladek)

While these concerns have become particularly compelling for hospitals under the new financial constraints of DRG-based reimbursement, they have in fact been recognized and acted upon by progressive hospitals well before the present era of prospective hospital reimbursement. Noteworthy in this regard is the long-standing home health care program for patients with chronic disease begun in 1947 at the Montefiore Medical Center (Bronx, New York), which has evolved to offer a wide array of other community-based rehabilitation and support services in the 1980s. This national prototype for hospital-sponsored community services, plus a series of case studies from other hospitals, all of which predate the DRG system, are described in *Hospitals and the Aged: The New Old Market* (Brody and Persily 1984).

The hospital's emerging role in community care of the elderly is currently the subject of a number of major initiatives on the part of hospital-related organizations and foundations throughout the country. Two particularly telling manifestations of the current surge of activity are, first, the development of a major multimillion dollar program entitled Hospital Initiatives in Long-Term Care, sponsored by the Robert Wood Johnson Foundation, and second, the recent creation by the American Hospital Association (A.H.A.) of a special section called Aging and Long-Term Care Services.

The Johnson Foundation program had, as of 1985, awarded sizable multiyear grants to 25 hospitals (selected from a pool of several hundred applicant institutions), with the stated primary objective "to encourage the development of model projects which will demonstrate that hospitals can develop comprehensive programs to better meet the health care needs of the elderly" (Robert Wood Johnson Foundation 1985, 914). The 25 awardees represent a diverse cross section of the nation's hospitals: 7 in rural settings, 9 major academic centers, 7 publicly owned, 5 multihospital consortia, 10 serving high proportions of minorities. Under the terms of the program, participating institutions are called upon to make available, in addition to existing acute care hospital services, certain nontraditional community-oriented services related to long-term care. The full set of terms of participation is shown in Appendix J. Central to all of the projects that have been developed are strong case management services to assure early identification of hospitalized elderly with long-term care needs and effective planning and coordination of community services to meet these needs. Through bringing about such changes in hospital services, the program seeks to impact in a measurable way the following two unmet or poorly met needs defined by the Johnson Foundation as "critical to promoting an acceptable quality of life for the aged": (1) the need for elderly persons to retain maximum independence and functional ability and to avoid unnecessary use of costly hospital and nursing home services; and (2) the need to improve the capabilities of physicians, nurses, and other hospital staff to care for the elderly in all areas of hospital activity, including emergency, outpatient, acute inpatient, and long-term care services.

The AHA Section on Aging and Long-Term Care Services has, in its several years in existence, sponsored a variety of efforts to inform and assist hospitals in addressing these needs. At the forefront of these activities has been a series of workshops on hospital-based case management services. In the view of many, this development represents an upgrading of the hospital's traditional discharge-planning activities, focusing with greater purpose on the particular posthospital needs of disabled elderly patients. While from the hospitals' point of view this development could be seen as a self-serving undertaking—expediting patient discharge and thereby avoiding the penalty imposed by DRG payment limitations—nonetheless this necessary, vigorous attention to discharge could allow hospitals to divert some of their vast material and professional resources to the largely neglected posthospital phase of patient well-being. In a provocative essay entitled "DRG: The second revolution in health care for the elderly," Brody and Magel (1984) argue that indeed the DRG-based reimbursement system is redefining the role of the hospital in ways that will lead to reallocation of acute care funds toward development of appropriate posthospital long-term support services, either directly provided by the hospital or through formalizing linkages with existing long-term care services. They see such developments particularly targeting that subgroup of elderly patients in need of what is referred to as "short-term long-term care" services. Figure 10-4, reproduced from this essay, demonstrates schematically the range of such services. Included among these are several modalities similar, if not identical, to those that have evolved earlier

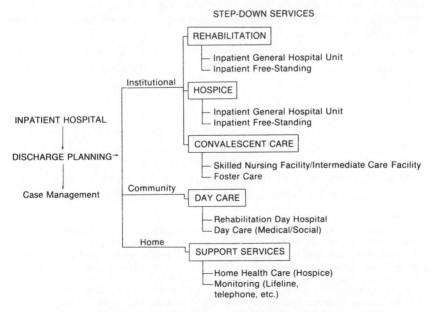

Figure 10-4 Model of a hospital-based system of short-term long-term care.
Source: Brody, S. J., and Magel. 1984. DRG—the second revolution in health care for the elderly. *Journal of American Geriatrics Society* 32:676–79. Reprinted with permission.

as part of British geriatrics services (e.g., the rehabilitation day hospital).*

Human Resources

The imperative for the medical profession to play a major role in delivering appropriate, high-quality care to the elderly is abundantly evident throughout the preceding sections of this book. The fact that this role has not been adequately fulfilled is equally evident in the form of numerous recent efforts to develop the research, educational, and service modes of the field, and perchance to develop the specialty of geriatric medicine in the United States (and other countries). The British experience clearly suggests that such explicit identification and commitment to the field of geriatric medicine has played an essential, though by no means singular, part in successful evolution of a continuum of services for the elderly. Recent U.S. experiences may be suitably reviewed from this point of view.

Research

Study of the aging process, the characteristics of disease in old age, and health services for the elderly have been of some identified interest to medical investigators in the United States since the beginning of the twentieth century when an American physician, Dr. I. L. Nascher, first coined the term *geriatrics*. The underlying principle of geriatric medicine was captured in an early piece of his writing on the subject: "The diseases of the aged are worthy of the most careful study. . . . *Let us not dismiss his ailments with the facile diagnosis: You are old*" (quoted in Penneton, Moritsugu, and Miller 1982; italics added). Little was heard from the field again until the 1930s and 1940s. In the late 1930s the U.S. Public Health Service established a center for gerontologic research which has flourished to this day and produced a formidable and unparalleled body of research on the normal aging process in man and animals (Shock et al. 1984). The 1940s saw the founding of the American Geriatrics Society and the Gerontological Society of America, the former mostly representing practicing physicians, the latter primarily representing academicians from

---

*While the logic of Brody and Magel's case is appealing, in the short run cost-containing strategies of HCFA have tended to thwart rather than support such developments, as summarized by Vladek in testimony before the Senate Special Committee on Aging hearings on the Prospective Payment System, 12 November 1985: "HCFA has impeded the granting of 2176 home and community-based care waivers to encourage the expansion of community-based long-term care services; has tried to gut quality of care standards for nursing homes; has arbitrarily narrowed the definition of 'skilled care' for Medicare home health benefits; and has recently proposed drastic cutbacks in reimbursement for covered home health services" (personal communication, 2 May 1986).

a number of disciplines concerned with health, social, psychological, economic, and other dimensions of aging. These societies publish major journals, sponsor annual scientific meetings, and undertake a variety of other educational, and increasingly public policy–oriented, activities. Research related to geriatrics received its greatest recognition with the founding of the National Institute on Aging in 1974. Under the leadership of Drs. Robert Butler (1974–1983) and T. Franklin Williams (1983–), the NIA has, through both intramural and extramural programs, encouraged research on a number of long-neglected specific health problems of the elderly (e.g., incontinence, gait problems and falling, osteoporosis, and particularly, dementia) as well as investigated fundamental biomedical, sociobehavioral, epidemiological, and health services problems related to aging and assessment of health status of elderly persons (NIA 1983). Of particular interest has been development of the concept of the Teaching Nursing Home, through which a number of academic medical centers affiliated with long-term care institutions have undertaken to develop active research and training programs targeted on problems of the chronically ill and disabled elderly (Butler 1981).*

Education and Training

In spite of long-standing recognition that the health problems of old age are important both for study and as a focus of national academic societies and journals, there has been a remarkable dearth of physician education or career development in the field. The failure of the field to develop as a medical specialty, analogous to pediatrics, is attributed to a lack of certain critical historical elements (Stevens 1977). The field clearly did not fit neatly into either of the two dominant trends in medical career development of the post–World War II era: the development of biomedical subspecialties, dominant from 1945 to 1970, and the trend toward primary care specialties from 1955 to 1980 (Maklan 1984). The American Medical Association physician masterfile for 1977 revealed that only 0.2 percent of responding physicians listed geriatrics as one of their principal areas of practice emphasis. These respondents tended to be considerably older, less likely to have any specialty certification, and less likely to belong to professional societies, as compared with all other respondents (Kane et al. 1980). Surveys of medical students and practicing physicians in the 1970s revealed little formal training and a generally negative attitude toward care of the elderly (Maklan 1984).

*A telephone survey of all academic medical centers in the country conducted by staff at the National Institute on Aging revealed that 90% have established formal academic affiliations with one or more nursing homes (personal communication, Marcia Ory, PRD, February 1987).

Facing this climate of medical noninvolvement, overshadowed by the clouds of high cost and questionable quality of hospital and nursing home care of the elderly, the United States has witnessed in the present decade a spate of vigorous initiatives to redress the gap in medical education and training in geriatrics and gerontology. These initiatives have recently been synthesized in a Symposium on the Geriatric Medical Education Imperative, sponsored by the New York Academy of Medicine (1985).

Among the first and potentially most significant initiatives was the publication and wide dissemination in 1978 of the Institute of Medicine (IOM) report on "Aging and Medical Education." After reviewing the extensive evidence of need for education in geriatrics in undergraduate and graduate medical education, the report primarily recommended that this be accomplished by faculty in preclinical and clinical departments developing new courses or integrating pertinent material into existing courses. A variety of such undertakings in fact ensued in response to state and federal grant support; however, relatively little substantial faculty or curriculum commitment to geriatrics in medical schools was evident five years later.* Reevaluating the situation in 1984, Dr. Paul Beeson, chairman for the 1978 IOM report, indicated his disappointment with what he referred to in retrospect as "the half-way measures that we recommended" and cited certain more fundamental requirements for the success of geriatrics as a medical discipline. These requirements included first his tentative endorsement of the development of independent academic departments of geriatric medicine. Such departments would have their own faculty and required curriculum, he reported, as does the prototype of such a department, established at Mount Sinai Medical Center in 1983. This approach has clearly had a major impact in strengthening geriatric medicine in Great Britain. Second, he pointed out the essential need for "a change in our system of health care payments whereby cognitive work and time spent in the care of people with chronic multiple disabilities is rewarded in a manner comparable to the rewards that come from carrying out procedures" Beeson 1985, 482).

In 1982 the Association of American Medical Colleges (AAMC), representing the nation's 127 medical schools as well as over 400 major teaching hospitals, conducted a series of four Regional Institutes on Geriatrics and Medical Education attended by deans and chairmen of major clinical and preclinical departments from over 90

*The number of medical schools with elective courses in geriatrics grew from 42 percent in 1977 to 66 percent in 1982–83 and 75 percent in 1983–84. However, on average, fewer than 4 percent of students were reported as actually taking an elective course or clerkship in geriatrics.

percent of the medical schools. The institutes, with the endorsement of this broad and influential constituency, arrived at a set of major recommendations with regard to supporting research and teaching, with particular emphasis on exposing students to problems and care modalities for the elderly in a variety of institutional and noninstitutional settings (Johnson 1985). The recommended physician's roles in care of elderly patients are strikingly different from the traditional biomedical model and in keeping with British precepts of geriatric medicine, as is evident in the section of recommendations entitled "Medical Management" reproduced in Appendix K.

The area of residency and fellowship training in geriatrics has developed in a more piecemeal fashion, compared with the aforementioned national consensus approaches to undergraduate medical education; however, to date, accomplishments at the postgraduate level appear to be more substantive, if modest in numbers. Having begun with 1 program and 2 positions in 1972, by 1984 in the United States there were a total of some 100 one- or two-year geriatric fellowship positions among 24 programs based in internal medicine departments and 13 programs in psychiatry and family medicine departments. Importantly, over half of the fellowships have been sponsored by the Veterans Administration, which has developed a series of Geriatric Research, Education, and Clinical Centers (GRECCs) based at major VA hospitals around the country. This development reflects the special need and available resources for providing for the large and rapidly aging population of veterans of World Wars I and II (see subsequent section "Comprehensive Services"). Other support for fellowships has come from the National Institute on Aging, Administration on Aging, and several private foundations. Recommendations for content and sites of training have been developed among fellowship programs. The majority of physicians completing the programs are assuming full-time roles in geriatric medicine, usually combining practice, teaching, and research (Libow and Cassel 1985). Little information is available to date to compare career styles of these contemporary entrants to geriatrics in the United States with their counterparts in Great Britain, as detailed in chapter 8.

The most recent major initiative related to personnel development is the "Report on Education and Training in Geriatrics and Gerontology" prepared by a committee of advisors convened by the NIA at the request of the House Committee on Appropriations. This comprehensive document reviews in detail the needs for personnel committed to the elderly from many other health and health-related fields in addition to medicine. Specific to medicine, the report calls for developing approximately 1,300 clinical faculty and a comparable number in basic sciences to adequately meet the needs of the nation's medical schools. At the time of that report only 250–300 such faculty were identified in the country (Williams 1985).

With movements now well under way to establish standards, faculty, and so forth for both undergraduate and postgraduate education, the debate over legitimizing geriatrics as a medical career is currently focused on the issue of specialty certification, or some variation thereof. To date, most of the national reports previously cited as well as the major medical specialties most readily associated with caring for the elderly (internal medicine, family medicine, psychiatry, rehabilitation medicine) have gone on record opposed to an independent specialty of geriatric medicine. While generally couched in terms of "the lack of a unique body of skills and knowledge," it seems clear that a more fundamental basis for such opposition is the competition such a new breed of specialist would pose. There has been more of a consensus in favoring a consultative role, mostly restricted to large hospital or nursing home settings. Acknowledging the importance of care of the elderly and the need to recognize those who pursue special training in this area, all of the previously mentioned fields have established special subcommittees, education task forces, and so forth to specify the particular needs of elderly patients to which their discipline should be attentive (Steel 1984). Among these groups, the American Board of Internal Medicine and the American Board of Family Practice have, as of 1985, submitted applications and received approval from the American Board of Medical Specialties to issue certificates of special competence in geriatrics to members of their specialty who have completed formal geriatrics fellowships or equivalent training (personal communication, Donald G. Langsley, 6 January 1986).

Service

In addition to the considerable movement afoot to establish research, undergraduate and postgraduate education, and professional credentials in the field of geriatric medicine, the development of new and nontraditional modes of medical practice is an essential final ingredient in the effective development of the field. In the absence of a prevalent practice model comparable to geriatric medicine units found throughout Great Britain, physicians practicing geriatric medicine in the United States tend to locate in a variety of settings that see fit to employ "a geriatrician." These range from academic and nonacademic hospitals and nursing homes, to health maintenance organizations or other forms of group practice, to solo fee-for-service practice. Within these various practice settings, a number of the essential tactics and strategies adapted by British geriatricians have begun to emerge in the United States.

Foremost among new modalities of medical practice are multi-disciplinary geriatric assessment or evaluation units (GAUs) in which physicians work in a collegial mode with various other health professionals concerned with rehabilitative and psychosocial problems of elderly persons. A recent survey identified a total of 126 GAUs in United States medical centers, 75 based at medical schools and 51 at Veterans Administration facilities. Fifty-three of these were inpatient services while 73 were ambulatory services (Epstein, Hall, and Besdine 1985). Examples of inpatient GAUs were discussed earlier in this chapter. Ambulatory units that have been described in detail include the prototype Evaluation-Placement project at Monroe Community Hospital (Williams et al. 1973) and its current successor at that hospital (Williams and Williams 1986), as well as units at Duke University (Moore et al. 1984) and the University of Pittsburgh (Martin et al. 1985). All of these ambulatory units link medical and psychiatric assessment with nursing, social, rehabilitative, and dietary assessment, and decisions about follow-up disposition are shared among the involved disciplines. The need for such a multidisciplinary approach is evident from the profile of medical diagnoses and related functional disorders among patients seen in a one-year period at the Monroe Community Hospital Geriatric Consultative Clinic, as summarized in table 10-2. This mode of geriatric medical practice, resembling that seen in British geriatric day hospitals,* has multiple objectives related to maximizing medical, physical, and social well-being of patient and care giver and avoiding unnecessary acute and chronic institutionalization. A randomized trial of the Consultative Clinic has shown a statistically significant reduction of hospital utilization and overall health care cost among persons referred to the program (personal communication, Mark Williams, March 1986).

The medical house call, a traditional mainstay of medical practice in Great Britain, but an almost lost component of medicine in the United States, is a second modality beginning to receive particular attention among physicians caring for the elderly in this country (Burton 1985). Various projects involving home visiting by physicians and other health professionals have reported improved diagnosis and management of elderly patients (Currie et al. 1981); evaluation of physical disabilities leading to successful rehabilitative interventions and environmental modifications (Liang et al. 1983); and medical, nursing, and social maintenance in the home among

*One recently described ambulatory geriatrics service, based at a community hospital in Los Angeles, has styled itself and named itself after the "British concept of the geriatric day hospital" (Morishita et al. 1986).

Table 10-2
Medical Conditions and Functional Difficulties among Persons Receiving
Evaluations in a Geriatric Consultative Clinic

	Number	Percent
Medical conditions		
Psychiatric disorders	59	45
Rheumatic disease	48	37
Dementing illness	42	32
Cardiovascular disease	41	31
Gastrointestinal disease	32	24
Hypertension	28	21
Pulmonary disease	22	17
Dermatologic disease	20	15
Renal disease	17	13
Other	37	28
Functional difficulties		
(moderate to severe)		
Bathing	59	46
Dressing	51	40
Toileting	30	24
Eating	33	26
Mobility	16	13
Handling money	84	65
Using telephone	50	29
Preparing food	86	68

Source: Adapted from Williams and Williams 1986. Reprinted with permission.

heavily dependent, sometimes terminally ill elderly persons (Brick-ner et al. 1975; Zimmer, Groth-Juncker, and McCusker 1985). The latter project has demonstrated in a randomized trial that a medically based home care program can significantly reduce institutionalization and overall cost while leading to a significantly higher level of satisfaction with care on the part of patients and their informal caretakers at home.

New approaches to medical care of nursing home residents have received considerable recent attention. In 1980 the American College of Physicians sponsored a conference on Changing Needs of Nursing Home Care, in recognition of the compelling need for internists to become more engaged in such care (American College of Physicians 1980). The conference reviewed several existing models of excellent medical care in nursing homes, but acknowledged that poor financial incentives and lack of attention to nursing homes in medical education and training pose formidable barriers to physician involvement in most situations. Among the several goals of the teaching nursing homes recently sponsored by the National Institute on Aging and several private foundations is the development of improved, progressive modes for providing medical care in nursing homes. The practice of the essentials of geriatric medicine, consisting of the provision of medical, psychiatric, rehabilitative, and custodial services by a multidisciplinary team, has been well described from the viewpoint of one prototypic teaching nursing home in New York (Libow 1982). Some teaching nursing homes have emphasized the potential role of gerontologic nurse practitioners, working with physicians, in providing day-to-day primary medical care of nursing home residents (Aiken et al. 1985). Such practice arrangements have been reported to provide high-quality care for nursing home residents in several settings (Kane et al. 1976; Kavesh, Mark and Kearney 1984; Wieland et al. 1986). This model seems particularly appropriate, first because of the relative dearth of physicians trained in geriatrics at the present and for the foreseeable future; second, and more important, because of the long tradition of the nursing profession in providing the continuous and comprehensive form of care that is particularly important among the chronically disabled residents of nursing homes.

Perhaps the most important attribute that distinguishes the practice of geriatric medicine from other clinical fields, and which is being explored in the United States, is physician involvement in mobilizing health and health-related resources, along with applying medical knowledge on behalf of elderly patients. In essence, geriatric medicine is in part a management role. This derives from the fact that providing for an individual's acute, rehabilitative, or long-term care needs may involve one or more of a variety of different hospital, community, or institutional staff and resources. Ideally the physician would be directly involved in the patient's care at whichever of these several levels and settings is required. Realistically this is not always feasible, nor necessarily appropriate. However, it is appropriate and essential, as exemplified in the British experience, for physicians caring for disabled elderly patients to be knowledgeable about the array of resources available and to collaborate actively in the process of care planning and follow-up for their patients. Certain distinguished medical leaders, while championing the cause of improved care for the elderly in the United States, have expressed reservations about physicians, "the most technologically specialized members of the team," becoming involved in such "case management" activities (Rogers 1983; Weksler, Durmaskin, and Kodner 1983). The question is framed as follows: "Should we encourage our most highly priced health professionals—physicians—who are best trained to handle acute, life threatening, biological events to become the organizers of the system?" (Rogers 1983, 124). To the extent that the role of medicine is restricted to "technological specialization" and "handling of acute life threatening biologic events," managerial activities would indeed be unsuitable. However, given that one's elderly patients are, as often as not, suffering from a complex of social, mental, and physical as well as biomedical problems, it is unrealistic, as those who practice geriatric medicine have found, to separate the medical treatment of the latter from the managerial aspects of the former. Physician participation in patient management should not be equated with dominance of the management role. But as implied, if not overtly stated in virtually all of the aforementioned position papers, surveys, and so forth, active physician involvement in multidisciplinary case management decisions is a high-priority, nontraditional role essential to the practice of geriatric medicine. In fact, as stated in chapters 4 and 5 and observed repeatedly in visiting geriatric services in Great Britain, the multidisciplinary case conference with vigorous physician participation is central to the effective and efficient practice of geriatric medicine.* This is in essence the British embodiment of "case management."

Comprehensive Services

The foregoing sections bear ample testimony to the fact that despite the fiscally and functionally fragmented state of health services for the elderly in the United States, some progressive initiatives have occurred. A number of these initiatives both enhance quality and reduce cost of care and frequently bear striking resemblance to components of the British system. However, as also noted, in the absence of a comprehensive system for financing and delivery of health services, these initiatives have commonly taken the form of special projects, demonstrations, waivers, or add-ons, acknowledged as worthy, but often destined to a limited or isolated existence. At best (or worst?) such innovations may, as in the instance of case management in its current highly publicized form, represent patchwork tactics introduced to more efficiently accommodate the elderly to the existing unplanned array of services.

By way of exception to such limitations, a small number of exemplary efforts to incorporate acute and chronic care for the elderly into one comprehensive organized service have in fact emerged in this country and may serve as models for others. Three distinctly different models may be discerned: (1) those instances in which enterprising traditional health care providers have through ingenuity pieced together existing Medicare, Medicaid, and related programs to create an ad hoc continuum of care for their elderly patients; (2) the systems

*Medical colleagues at the City Hospital Department of Geriatric Medicine in Edinburgh considered the weekly multidisciplinary case conference at which the status and treatment/management plans for all active inpatients (thirty-five to forty patients) was reviewed to be the most important two hours of the week.

developed by some Veterans Administration medical centers, linking together their existing facilities and personnel; and (3) those comprehensive care systems that have evolved from the health maintenance organization prepaid model of health service delivery.

An Ad Hoc Continuum of Services

Creative efforts of individuals and institutions have in a number of situations woven together various separately organized and separately reimbursed health service modalities to arrive at consolidated, comprehensive systems of care for frail elderly persons. Two notable examples of this phenomenon, one in Cleveland, Ohio (Frengeley 1985), the other in Milwaukee, Wisconsin (Fisk 1983), have developed from acute hospitals. In each instance, a strong commitment from the hospital's executive-administrative level, combined with the fortuitous close proximity and effective affiliation with an inpatient rehabilitation facility and the presence of strong medical and multidisciplinary professional leadership, formed the nidus for organizing comprehensive geriatrics services. Both programs have developed ambulatory services providing primary medical care and special geriatric assessment clinics. Strong linkages with home health services and one or more nursing homes have been established, and one of the programs (Milwaukee) includes a rehabilitation-oriented day hospital modeled after the British prototypes. Both programs provide their array of organizationally linked services to elderly patients from the surrounding urban communities in which they are located. Services are reimbursed through traditional Medicare, Medicaid, and private out-of-pocket mechanisms, plus significant special developmental grant monies. These experiences, emanating from hospitals that have a vivid picture of unmet needs of elderly patients, are reminiscent of the origins of some geriatric units in Great Britain. One limitation is the lack of a clear definition of the populations served, which is important in planning type and amount of services needed. With a view to this and related concerns, it has been proposed that such hospital-based comprehensive programs evolve into prepaid plans, with defined populations such as discussed subsequently (Fisk 1983).

In Boston a continuum of health services for chronically ill elderly persons was organized in 1977 by a small nonprofit group practice of salaried primary care physicians known as the Urban Medical Group. In this program, the founding physician group assumed responsibility for full medical care for some 3,000 ambulatory, 280 homebound, and 360 nursing home–based elderly persons. Providing care for patients in each of these settings as well as in the acute hospital when needed was facilitated by employing nurse practitioners and physician assistants to work in primary care teams with the physicians. Reimbursement, while coming largely from Medicare and Medicaid, included certain special waivers for reimbursing the nurse practitioners and physician assistants. This organized approach to care at several levels has led to cost savings through lower use of nursing home and acute hospital care and higher use of home care services than seen in comparison settings (Master et al. 1980). At this writing, negotiations are in progress to evolve the financing of this program into a prepayment mode, combining Medicare and Medicaid funds (personal communication, William Kavesh, December 1985).*

The On Lok Community Care Organization for Dependent Adults, located in San Francisco, is a consolidated care system developed specifically to serve older patients with established functional dependencies and long-term care needs. The program evolved from a multipurpose neighborhood day care center in the early 1970s to become a comprehensive system of medical and social services for dependent elderly persons by the early 1980s, as illustrated in figure 10-5. The driving forces behind this development were on the one hand a growing population of dependent elderly and on the other hand a relative scarcity of traditional long-term care (nursing home) resources to meet their needs. This prompted the On Lok staff to develop a single service system to meet the full range of possible medical and social needs of its constituency and a mechanism for funding it. The latter was achieved through an unusual set of Medicare waivers that allowed pooling of public and private funds to establish prepaid capitated financing for all medical, rehabilitative, and social services, delivered in both inpatient and outpatient settings and utilizing the most suitable resources. The resulting system provides a broad array of services emphasizing noninstitutional modalities, as shown in figure 10-5. This approach, which resembles the comprehensive system of geriatrics services found in Great Britain, has been achieved at per capita costs that are substantially lower than those in the traditional discontinuous approach to providing acute and long-term care services in the United States (Zawadski and Ansak 1983).†

---

*Beginning in 1987, "Medicap," a communitywide program in Monroe County, New York, analogous in purpose to the Boston Urban Medical Group program, will undertake to organize and finance the full continuum of acute, sub-acute, and long-term care services (including full nursing home stays) for the entire population (some 9,000) of persons over age 65 who are or become Medicaid eligible. In this unique program, sponsored by a waiver grant from the Health Care Financing Administration, Medicare and Medicaid funds will be pooled and a prepaid, capitated sum will be paid to the program for each enrollee (personal communication, James Fatula, January 1987).

†Because of its demonstrated success in providing a comprehensive and efficient program of services for dependent elderly persons, the On Lok program has had its waiver status extended indefinitely (U.S. Public Law 99-272, 99th Cong., 7 April 1986).

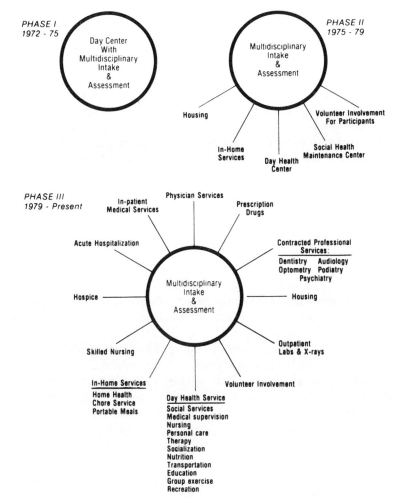

Figure 10-5 On Lok's health program development, 1972–81.
Source: Zawadski, R. T. and Ansak, M. L. 1983. Consolidating community-based long-term care: Early returns from the On Lok demonstration. *The Gerontologist* 23:364–69. Reprinted with permission.

The Veterans Administration

The Veterans Administration was created by an act of Congress in 1946 to consolidate and extend a series of service programs for a large and growing population of veterans of the two world wars. Included

Also in 1986 the Robert Wood Johnson Foundation established a grant program to assist a number of other sites in the country to develop similar prepaid comprehensive long-term care programs in consultation with the On Lok staff (personal communication, Bruce Friedman, Monroe County Long-Term Care Program, July 1986).

among these programs were old age homes, which were originally developed for veterans of the Civil War, and a series of general hospitals built following the two world wars. In the 1950s, services at some of the hopsitals were broadened to include intermediate medical care units for convalescing patients. In 1973 a number of hospital-based home care programs were established to provide medical, nursing, and rehabilitative assistance to homebound patients and their care givers in the community. Most recently, since the late 1970s, inpatient and outpatient geriatric evaluation units have been established at over forty-five VA medical centers. In the long-term care area, a nursing home program was officially established in 1979. Given availability of these resources, combined with the rapid increase in numbers of aging veterans entitled to medical care, the Veterans Administration has in recent years made a strong commitment to fashioning progressive geriatrics services. This has been manifested most vividly through establishment of eight Geriatric Research, Education, and Clinical Centers with the mission of training physicians in geriatric medicine and conducting research into ways to best meet the medical care needs of the elderly. As part of this resource development strategy, the VA has also emphasized linking together various components of its services into a continuum of care options for its patients. Foremost among these "structural" developments has been the widespread implementation of multidisciplinary geriatric evaluation units (GEUs) that link acute care with rehabilitation and appropriate posthospital placement and care (Mather and Abel 1986). This concept, which embodies the essential features of hospital-based geriatric units in Great Britain, has been strongly encouraged throughout the VA system, following reports of the striking effectiveness of GEUs in Sepulveda and elsewhere, as reviewed earlier in this chapter (VA chief medical director's letter, "Geriatric Evaluation Unit," 2 February 1983).

While largely restricted to meeting health care needs of elderly males, nevertheless the organizational accomplishments of the VA geriatrics services, existing under one broad administration and budget, have in many ways emulated accomplishments of district geriatrics services developed under the British National Health Service. As testimony to the achievements of the VA programs, two national conferences on organized health services for the frail elderly have been jointly sponsored by the VA and the American Health Planning Association. Proceedings of the first of these have been published in a monograph entitled *The Complex Cube of Long Term Care* (Oriol 1985).

Health Maintenance Organizations

In its quest for cost-containment strategies in the 1980s, the Medicare program has in a stepwise fashion explored the role of health maintenance organizations in care of the elderly. Following the successful experience of five demonstration projects in which HMOs provided high-quality care to elderly enrollees for prepaid premiums of 95 percent of the average community cost per person under Medicare, prepaid plans became an official Medicare option as part of the Tax Equity and Fiscal Responsibility Act of 1982. In response to this opportunity, over one hundred HMOs have since entered risk-based programs for enrolling and serving Medicare patients (Iglehart 1985).

While principally promoted for achieving efficient delivery of the acute physician and hospital services traditionally covered by the Medicare program, HMO involvement in care of large numbers of elderly persons, many of whom have chronic diseases or disabilities, has of necessity led to the introduction of a number of nontraditional care modalities. Such service innovations, which are fully feasible under the flexible terms upon which an HMO is able to deploy its budget, have primarily focused upon avoiding hospital admissions or preventing administrative delays in discharge from hospital. Exemplary in this regard are the array of "continuing care" service innovations developed by one HMO, with which I am directly acquainted, during its first two years in serving a population of 5,000–6,000 Medicare enrollees. These innovations include establishing full-time social work and discharge planning programs within the major hospital to which HMO patients are admitted; contracting with the local visiting nurse service for prompt seven-day-a-week provision of a wide variety of skilled and unskilled home support services; establishing linkage with a rehabilitation-oriented skilled nursing facility to ease transfer of hospitalized patients; identifying one physician as having overall responsibility for the ongoing medical care of elderly plan members residing in nursing homes (Worden 1985).*

As an effective way to provide acute and subacute medical care for the elderly, the Medicare-HMO programs appear successful. However, the services described above are relatively short term in duration, relating ultimately to episodes of acute care. True continuing care (long-term care) in community or institution remains a major uncovered service in these programs and a challenge being met by cur-

*A study of the evolution of these continuing care services, their utilization, and impact is in progress. On initial review, there are striking resemblances to many of the elements in the continuum of services for the elderly, found in a British health district (Barker 1986a).

rent explorations,* the most advanced of which is the "social health maintenance organization."

Social Health Maintenance Organizations

In the Deficit Reduction Act of 1984 (P.L. 98-36) Congress directed the Secretary of Health and Human Services to demonstrate the concept of a social health maintenance organization. . . . This unusual action reflects strong national interest in finding new delivery systems for the elderly that have the potential to be cost-effective as well as comprehensive. More important, it indicates that national leaders recognize the inevitable and growing mismatch between the need for care resulting from demographic trends and the ability of the public sector to provide the necessary resources. This imbalance demands new approaches and ideas. (Leutz et al. 1985, xi)

The launching of the social health maintenance organization (SHMO) represents a uniquely American quest for a fiscally and organizationally sophisticated true continuum of health and health-related services for the chronically ill elderly. On the one hand the SHMO draws on the prepayment, risk-sharing insurance principle whereby health maintenance organizations have provided high-quality traditional and nontraditional medical care to enrolled populations within a fixed budget (Luft 1981). On the other hand, it extends this system of prepaid shared risk to include provision of chronic as well as acute care services to elderly enrollees. In so doing, the developers of the SHMO concept at the Brandeis University Health Policy Center have begun to address three fundamental problems of health services for the elderly in the United States. First is the lack of an adequate policy for insuring against the costs of long-term care, in contrast to the existence of strong insurance against costs of acute medical care. Second is the separation and lack of coordination between acute and chronic care services at both institutional and professional levels. Third, and closely related to the first two problems, is the lack of reimbursement incentives for providers in the acute and chronic care sectors to seek efficient and innovative ways to meet the multifaceted care needs of the chronically ill elderly (Leutz et al. 1985, ch. 1).

*InterStudy, a non-profit health care research firm, the country's leading source of studies of the development and performance of HMOs, has recently instituted a Center for Aging and Long-Term Care which is undertaking several initiatives in 1987 to identify and promote innovative approaches for integrating acute and long-term care in Medicare HMOs (personal communication, Laura Iversen, InterStudy, 3 February 1987).

Following several years of planning and development, supported by a number of private foundations, and the passage of the 1984 authorizing legislation, four sites embarked on the SHMO experiment in 1985. An overview of these four organizationally diverse and geographically dispersed sites is provided in table 10-3. Each site is charged to enroll a cross section of elderly members whose payments are covered from a pool of Medicare and Medicaid funds, supple-

Table 10-3
Overview of SHMO Demonstration Sites

Site Sponsor	Type of Sponsor	Relationship to Partner	Key Opportunities and Obstacles
Metropolitan Jewish Geriatric Center, Brooklyn, N.Y. (Elderplan, Inc.)	Comprehensive chronic care agency	Capitation contract and risk sharing with small affiliated medical group. Community hospital contracted on per diem basis.	*Opportunity:* large untapped market *Obstacle:* creating an HMO and medical group
Kaiser Permanente Medical Care Program, Portland, Oreg. (Medicare Plus II)	Large established HMO	No partners— SHMO added to existing Kaiser system	*Opportunity:* use experience and reputation *Obstacle:* creating LTC services
Ebenezer Society, Minneapolis, Minn. (Medicare Partners)	Comprehensive chronic care agency	Partnership agreement with large established HMO for all acute medical care. Bottom-line risk sharing	*Opportunity:* expertise and image of partners *Obstacle:* competitive HMO market
Senior Care Action Network, Long Beach, Calif. (SCAN Health Plan, Inc.)	Case management/brokerage agency	Separate contracts with established medical group and medical center hospital. Both on capitation/risk basis	*Opportunity:* large untapped market *Obstacle:* management and incentives in the system

Source: Greenberg et al. 1985. Reprinted with permission.

mented by private out-of-pocket contributions. Details of organizational, operational, and fiscal aspects of the project as a whole, and for
each of the four sites, are contained in a monograph prepared by the
professional staff at Brandeis University (Leutz et al. 1985).

Of greatest interest from the perspective of the present book is the
section of the Brandeis monograph subtitled "Creating a Continuum
of Care," which elaborates the core package of acute and chronic care
services to be offered by all sites. These services include unlimited
acute hospital days and medical visits without copayments or deduct-
ibles, plus coverage for many specific items such as dentures, eye-
glasses, hearing aides, podiatry, preventive visits, prescription
drugs, and so forth. Core chronic care benefits include case management, home nursing and therapies, homemaker services, day care,
transportation, hospice care, home-delivered meals, and limited
amounts of skilled and custodial care in nursing homes. (A detailed
chart of SHMO benefits compared with traditional limited Medicare
benefits is contained in Appendix I.) Delivery system components to
accommodate the array of benefits are shown schematically in figure
10-6. The physical locations of the various components vary according to the local circumstances of each site; for example, the day care
center may be attached to a hospital, nursing home, or community
agency. By comparison, this full spectrum of service common to each
SHMO, with local variations in physical configuration, is reminiscent of the local variations on the similar common theme of providing
a continuum of services which was noted among the British geriatric
medicine services discussed in chapter 5.

Professional staffing and division of labor in meeting the broad
commitments to its subscribers pose a particular challenge to the
SHMO model. As discussed in the monograph by Leutz et al. (1985),
the key providers to be considered are the medical and case management staff. Physicians will be called upon to deal with a patient
population with complex problems, many of which are best addressed
by care modalities (preventive, rehabilitative, educational, social)
with which they have often had little experience in medical training
and practice. Significant time will be required to work with other
professionals in a multidisciplinary team modality in developing
care plans and consulting on an ad hoc basis with nurse practitioners
and others involved in actually providing much of the care to patients
in home or nursing home settings. Clearly these activities are very
similar to the work of the British consultant in geriatric medicine,
and appropriately, the SHMO developers speculate on the need to
recruit or train physicians with special geriatrics skills.

The principal role and challenge for case management will be

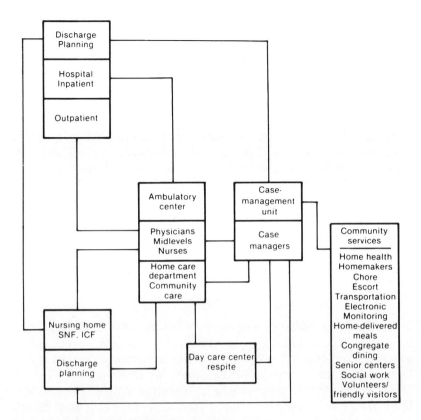

Figure 10-6 SHMO service delivery components.
Source: Leutz, W. N.; Greenberg, J. N.; and Abrahams, R. et al. 1985. *Changing Health Care for an Aging Society.* Lexington, Mass.: D.C. Heath. Reprinted with permission.

presiding over utilization of long-term care resources in a manner that both assures quality care and operates within budgetary limits. In this role it is expected that case managers will work closely with direct service providers in assessing client need for long-term care services and in planning and monitoring use of such services. The case manager will ultimately control resource utilization by acting as the official authorizing agent for approving long-term care services. Many issues regarding eligibility, targeting, and establishment of norms for chronic care services are being explored in the implementation of these case management aspects of the SHMO (Leutz et al. 1985, ch. 4).* As noted earlier in discussing case management, one

*In assessing this issue under the subtopic "professionals or bureaucrats for case managers?" in a recent study, Walter Leutz of the Brandeis University Health Policy

finds in the British geriatrics service that clinical assessment and management decisions regarding service modalities are largely carried out in concert on the part of direct service providers, without the addition of an independent case management function. A similar approach to case management has developed among physicians and their associates in the On Lok and Urban Medical Group comprehensive geriatrics services described earlier (Leutz et al. 1985, 70). It remains to be seen how the SHMO projects will resolve the question of independence versus close continuity between clinical and case management functions. There is reason for concern that an independent case management entity could become excessively concerned with enforcing eligibility criteria and other forms of constraint over service utilization in the interest of fiscal accountability, analogous to past experiences with Medicare benefits. Such a turn of events would seriously detract from the otherwise highly attractive SHMO comprehensive care concept.

Summary

In the face of rapidly escalating expenditures for acute and long-term care under the Medicare and Medicaid programs, respectively, a number of major policy proposals for reforming the organization and financing of health services for the elderly have been developed in the 1980s. None of these proposals has been acted upon at the national level. However, a number of important elements of organized geriatrics services similar to those observed in Great Britain have recently been introduced in the United States through special projects. These health service developments include strategies for incorporating geriatric rehabilitation into acute hospitals, initiatives for improving the quality of both rehabilitation services and acute medical care for residents of nursing homes, and an extensive series of projects for providing community-based alternatives to nursing home placement for elderly patients who require long-term care. Additionally, leaders in both undergraduate and graduate medical education have begun explicitly to incorporate geriatric medicine into medical school curriculum and postgraduate fellowship training programs and to establish certification for specialty training. Finally, and most gratifying, a number of model approaches to delivering a comprehensive continuum of health care for the elderly have been

---

Center reaches the following conclusion: "The professional model (along the lines of the physician) seems more appropriate for assessing and making decisions based on the complex mixes of physical, social, and economic factors that surround long-term care cases" (Leutz 1986, 138).

developed within the United States. The most recent and perhaps most advanced of these emerging models is the social health maintenance organization. Given these pragmatic, but as yet tentative, developments in response to the geriatric imperative in the United States, it is incumbent upon health policy makers to work toward establishing a national health program that firmly supports such developments as part of the mainstream of health services in this country.

CHAPTER 11

Conclusion

Twice-Told Tales

I have no doubt that the great energy and inventiveness of American medicine, freed of the shackles of traditional models of health care which are no longer appropriate, will rise to these challenges.
—J. WILLIAMSON, 1987

At the end of the nineteenth century in both Great Britain and the United States, the old and disabled person of limited means was at risk of ending his or her days in a poorhouse. Those who could afford care in the home avoided such a fate—and avoided admission to a hospital as well. Medical technology was limited to what was contained in a doctor's bag.

During the twentieth century, the populations of both countries have experienced comparable demographic and epidemiologic transitions, resulting in increasingly aging populations in which chronic diseases constitute the dominant health problems (Grundy 1983). Concurrently, delivery of medical care has undergone dramatic changes accompanied by strikingly different organizational patterns in Great Britain and the United States. Of the many profound consequences of these divergent developments, perhaps none is more striking than the differences in organization and mix of services provided to care for the elderly with chronic disease: the British National Health Service delivering a comprehensive, organizationally linked spectrum of preventive, curative, rehabilitative, and supportive care; the pluralistic, privately owned, publicly regulated U.S. health care system giving rise to fragmented services with little explicit provision for a continuum of care.

An excellent analysis of the economic, political, social, and cultural forces accounting for development of the respective health care systems in Great Britain and the United States has recently been published (Hollingsworth 1986) and will not be pursued here. Rather, the present study describes and contrasts the evolution of health services for the elderly within the two systems and considers the potential applicability of the British experience in the United States. I contend, with a measure of optimism, that in spite of major differences in ownership, organization, and financing health services in the two countries, strategies and tactics for providing comprehensive health care for the elderly which have evolved so successfully in Great Britain do have exportable features and that these are strongly to be commended to the United States. Others have made comparative observations of this issue from various perspectives in recent years. A brief review of their writings reveals a general consensus very much in line with the conclusions to be drawn from the present study.

In a short essay entitled "Care of the Aged: An English Lesson?" published in 1974, two community medicine physicians interested in studying the effect of national approaches to health care financing on the practice of clinical medicine focus on care of the frail elderly as a case in point (Smits and Draper 1974). They concentrate in particular on the evolution of specialized hospital-based geriatrics units within the National Health Service framework, describing this development as "a support service for the general practitioner that is a model of health care, centered on the patient and the overall population rather than on an organ and its diseases" (p. 747). The incorporation of rehabilitation and psychiatry into geriatric medicine, alongside of the usual clinical skills of internal medicine and the fact that "geriatricians are by necessity coordinators and collaborators in multispecialty teams" (p. 747), are emphasized. By contrast, the authors review the narrowly medicalized terms of care of the frail elderly which had evolved in the United States and been reinforced under the terms of the Medicare program, as discussed in chapter 9. Written at a time when several proposals for national health insurance were being seriously entertained in this country, the authors intended in part to recommend evolution of American health care financing toward a broader form of coverage conducive to development of comprehensive geriatrics services such as seen in Great Britain.

In another essay written in the mid-1970s, "Geriatric Care in the United Kingdom: An American Perspective," health policy analyst Anne Somers (1976) focuses on approaches to long-term care needs. Of particular interest to her is British emphasis on care in the community, with extensive provision for medical, nursing, and social services in the home as well as the use of day hospitals and intermittent respite admission to institutions. These developments are contrasted with the more costly and less appropriate reliance upon nursing homes for long-term care and conspicuous dearth of provision for

community-based services in the United States. While favorably disposed to the British approach, Somers points out the imperative, in
her view, for such community-oriented services to become more involved in "preventive geriatrics" as the demand for long-term care
increased with the aging of populations. Such practices have, as discussed in chapter 7, gained increasing attention in Great Britain over
the past decade.* In this regard, the contribution of community nurse
attachments in general practices is particularly stressed in a more
recent essay on British community services for the elderly by another
American health policy analyst (Zwick 1985).

An in-depth comparison of care of elderly patients in long-term
care institutions in Britain and the United States was conducted by
an American nurse-anthropologist Jeanie Schmit Kayser-Jones early in the 1980s. Published in a monograph, *Old, Alone, and Neglected*
(1981), and several companion papers, her participant-observer studies of a continuing care institution in Scotland and a skilled nursing
facility in the United States reveal markedly higher-quality social,
nursing, and medical care as well as staff morale in the former. In
explaining the differences between the two societies in the long-term
care setting, the author briefly reviews the well-developed strategies
for meeting needs of elderly at all stages of a continuum of care in
Britain (as detailed in the present study) and points out the essential
structural factors that have facilitated such developments there, but
have been lacking in the United States. These in her view include a
comprehensive government insurance program, training of medical
specialists in care of the elderly, and a successful linking together of
geriatrics services to provide for continuing, comprehensive care
(1982). In their critical analysis, *The Nursing Home in American
Society,* Johnson and Grant (1985) reiterate these points in a brief
section that begins by acknowledging that "most reformers look to
Great Britain for innovations in the care of the elderly" (p. 157).

A monograph entitled *Geriatric Medicine in the United States and
Great Britain* (Carboni 1982) provides a sophisticated sociological
analysis of the contrasting circumstances that led to successful development of geriatrics as a medical specialty in Great Britain, but
failed to do so in the United States. The author cites the essential role

---

*Interestingly, as British health services in the community moved beyond long-
term supportive care and toward a preventive geriatrics mode in the latter 1970s and
1980s, a variety of community-oriented demonstration projects also began to appear in
the United States. However, the latter consisted almost entirely of long-term care
alternatives to institutionalization, with minimal emphasis on preventive or rehabilitative services. Comparison of these strategies as reflections of the two different
health care systems is provided in a study contrasting developments in Edinburgh
(Scotland) and Rochester (New York) (Barker 1985).

of the National Health Service Act in leading to the development of hospital-based geriatrics services, staffed by consultant physicians (see ch. 3). Given such a clearly defined existence, including alloca- tion of health service resources (although comparatively meager in the formative years), geriatric medicine attained the necessary "power" base and unambiguous identity considered a prerequisite for developing a medical specialty. This development was followed by establishment of academic departments and professorships and de- ployment of medical students and postgraduate trainees to geriatrics services in general hospitals, as detailed in chapter 8. By contrast, Carboni points out the pluralism of medical roles subsumed under the aegis of geriatrics in the United States, with the greatest barrier to specialty status being the lack of allocation of resources, compara- ble to the British geriatrics unit, with which to give "collective identi- ty" to the field. This critical void in U.S. health services has been maintained both by professional barriers on the part of established specialties (primarily internal medicine, family medicine, and psy- chiatry) whose "turf" would be encroached upon by geriatrics ser- vices and by the fee-for-service mode of physician reimbursement which does not adequately compensate for the patient-intensive (as opposed to technology-intensive) mode of geriatric care. The author does note, however, by the early 1980s several exceptions to this state of affairs had begun to appear, hence introducing opportunities and incentives for explicit geriatrics services and careers in the United States; these exceptions are the Veterans Administration Geriatric Centers and the initial involvements of health maintenance organi- zations in enrolling Medicare recipients on a prepaid basis (Carboni 1982, ch. 7). Indications are that those geriatrics service modalities that have since evolved in such settings in the United States (see ch. 10) have drawn heavily on prototypes on the opposite side of the Atlantic. Furthermore, as in Britain, academic status in the form of professorships and required medical school curriculum has begun to be accorded geriatric medicine, as have standards for certifying those with postgraduate training in the field. These developments fulfill the forecast offered by another interested American physician after visiting Great Britain several years ago: "If American geriatrics does flourish in the coming years, it will be largely because of the stimulus of the British example" (Campion 1980).*

---

*As a case in point, Dr. William Hazzard (1986), Chairman of the Department of Medicine in Bowman Gray School of Medicine, has recently undertaken a department- wide initiative in gerontology and geriatrics. In embarking upon this experiment he acknowledges the importance of a sabbatical in Great Britain: "I continue to gain resolve and inspiration from the examples of my colleagues in the United Kingdom, my continuing Ode to British geriatrics" (p. 311).

Important elements—tactics, strategies—of British geriatrics services in the community, the hospital, the long-term care institu tion, along with development of medical personnel, have been extensively described and examined in these pages and in those of other observers. They are summarized in table 11-1. The frequent absence of these elements from traditional health services in the United States, but more important, their evident applicability and successful initial adaptation in selected situations in this country, has been noted. The further evolution, documentation, and evaluation of such developments in the United States is to be commended. Toward this end, a list of recommendations for research and development related to specific elements in the continuum of health services for the elderly is provided in Appendix L.

While the various elements listed in table 11-1 are necessary in one form or other to provide comprehensive care for the elderly, they are not on their own sufficient. Witness the shortcomings of hospital-based geriatrics projects that lack community follow-up components and of community-based long-term care demonstrations developed independent of existing medical services; witness the frequent failure of nursing homes, developed and operated outside of the mainstream of medical services, to provide rehabilitative or primary

Table 11-1

Some Specific Elements of Comprehensive Health Services for the Elderly in Great Britain

Community	*General Hospital,* continued
Enrollment in primary care	Liaison consultation with other
practice	hospital services
—General practitioner	—Medicine
—Attached community nurses	—Orthopedics
—Home visiting by GPs and	—Psychiatry
nurses	*Institutional Continuing Care*
Social service liaisons	Geriatric assessment and re-
—Home helps	habilitation prior to admission
—Meals-on-wheels	Medical surveillance: avoid fre-
—Domiciliary occupational	quent transfer to hospital
therapy	Multidisciplinary rehabilitation:
General Hospital	maintenance of function
Acute geriatrics services	Social and recreational activities
—Defined catchment population	*Education*
for referrals	Academic departments of geriatric
—Geriatric medicine specialists,	medicine
house staff	Required curriculum in medical
—Multidisciplinary teams	schools
—Rehabilitation emphasis	Formal postgraduate specialty
—Home visiting	training
—Day hospital	Postgraduate training for primary
—Respite admissions	care practitioners

medical care effectively, and other examples discussed in chapters 9 and 10. Rather, in the end one must give equal if not greater attention to the organizational structure of the health care system within which the elements are knit together, and specifically ask *What are the prospects for such structural reform in the United States?* In answering this question, it is helpful to refer to the thoughtful reflections of several leading scholars from the social sciences.

In 1975 the American medical sociologist David Mechanic advanced the thesis that the convergence of several major challenges to medical services common to modern nations would ultimately lead to the convergence of approaches to medical care organization. In developing this thesis he emphasized that "all medical care systems, like other social institutions, develop within their own historical circumstances and forms of professional organization, and thus the hypothesis of convergence does not imply that they develop identical patterns of organization. It does argue, however, that they all strive to deal with certain common problems and, in coping with these in the most effective way, they become more similar" (p. 241). The common experiences he perceives in modern nations in the later part of the twentieth century include increased tendencies to reduce inequalities in access to health care and to provide health services to defined communities or populations; the quest for integration of fragmented components of health services; the quest for adequate primary medical care resources; and the need to develop such services more efficiently in response to cost escalations. To these may be added the related thoughts of Thomas McKeown (1973), a leading figure in the field of social medicine in Great Britain, who sees the clash between two historic trends—the increasing importance of chronic disease and disability associated with aging and the alarming advance in very costly medical technology—constituting an imperative to reconsider the traditional organization of medical services in industrialized societies: "Serious mistakes in organization will be penalized more heavily than in the past, and it is therefore essential to devise a new pattern in accord with the character of the residual health problems and the trend in medical technology" (p. 19).*

In the final chapter of his widely acclaimed study, *The Social*

*Convergence of health care systems for the elderly toward organized programs with elements in common with the British experience in fact does appear to be occurring in a number of other industrialized nations. Specifically, Canada and other British Commonwealth nations have begun in recent years to adopt the concept of geriatric medicine as a specialty concerned with presiding over and orchestrating services for care of the frail elderly (personal communication, Dr. Ronald Cape, 16 September 1985). The leadership in such instances has generally come from physicians who have taken formal training in geriatric medicine in Great Britain. That countries outside the British sphere are similarly evolving integrated services, tailored to the health

Transformation of American Medicine, Paul Starr (1982) sets the scene of emerging patterns of health care delivery in the United States. Starr finds that, following roughly a century of sovereignty of the medical profession in determining the structure and content of the country's medical services, control has passed to corporate organizations. While reflecting a societal response to varying degrees to all of Mechanic's and McKeown's converging forces, the corporate approach to organizing and operating health services is preeminently a response to the challenge to achieve efficiency in a fragmented field that has become dominated by cost concerns. Central to each of the several emerging models of corporate health care that Starr discusses—academic medical center networks, nonprofit and for-profit multihospital systems, health maintenance organizations serving defined populations, and diversified health care "conglomerates" which do not serve defined populations—is the principle of integration of resources for purposes of effective and efficient, hence competitive, delivery of health services.

The integration of resources on the part of the various models of corporate health care hold very different implications for development of comprehensive health services for the elderly. Among the less promising are both the academic networks, whose objectives are primarily to assure viable arrangements for their traditional biomedically oriented education and research interests, and the "horizontally integrated" multihospital systems, wherein the principal objective is to reduce competition and achieve economies of scale through capturing large sectors of the traditional acute care hospital sector. Little structural reform toward forging links between acute and chronic care services is implied by these two strategies. By contrast, the "vertical integration" of multiple health service modalities (hospital, home care, nursing home, other) characteristic of the "diversified conglomerate" model and the health maintenance organiza-

---

care needs of the elderly, is exemplified in the following statements from Denmark and Japan.

From a special issue of the *Danish Medical Bulletin:* "The justification for the existence of a separate specialty in LTM (long term medicine) is that the total care of old people cannot be carried out within the normal system by which internal medicine is practised. Whilst first and foremost a clinician, the geriatrician has special interests which include physical rehabilitation, the management of the day hospital, the encouragement of a preventive service, the overall development within a given area of a total medical service for the elderly and the management of long term care" (Dalgaard 1982, 132).

From a speech presented by the head of Social Security Section of the Institute of Public Health in Japan, addressing that country's dilemma with escalating costs of medical care of the aged: "It will be necessary to reorganize health and human service resources. This reorganization should be based on the principle of comprehensive, coordinated community based alternatives to institutionalized care" (Maeda 1985, 12).

tion model represents structural changes that are clearly conducive to developing a continuum of services for the elderly. These models may in fact be seen as playing a role roughly analogous to the critical role played by district health authorities of the British National Health Service in consolidating acute and chronic care under one administrative mechanism.

In pursuing the analogy, it is instructive to note the extent to which certain essential organizational features of British health services may be attained in the United States. These features include (1) a prospectively determined budget for personal health services, and (2) responsibility for a defined population, both of which provide incentives to plan efficient coordinated use of resources, and (3) a commitment to provide comprehensive health services to the population served. The aforementioned "diversified conglomerate" lacks the first two criteria and may or may not pursue development of comprehensive health services as a principal objective. Health maintenance organizations and related prepaid delivery systems, however, do clearly fulfill the first two criteria of serving a defined population under a prospectively determined budget. While primarily promoted as part of national health policy for containing rising costs of personal health services, HMOs and other prepaid medical plans have also in principle been committed to providing comprehensive health care in order to appeal to prospective members. Not surprisingly then, as discussed at the end of chapter 10 and elsewhere (Bonano and Wetle 1984), a number of emerging comprehensive programs for providing care to the elderly in the United States have either evolved into or evolved from prepaid health care delivery systems. In so doing they have begun to incorporate various of the elements of organized geriatrics services listed in table 11-1. That such developments are possible and highly desirable, but will require continued concerted efforts, is eloquently articulated in several recent reviews of the role of prepaid delivery systems in chronic care (Bonano and Wetle 1984; Knickman and McCall 1986; Schlesinger 1986). Obstacles to be overcome include attitudinal and institutional barriers to dealing with chronic disease as well as uncertainties in estimating costs and assuring quality in providing chronic care to elderly enrollees. These are certainly surmountable.

In summary, a capacity for introducing innovative health care modalities responsive to the particular needs of elderly persons has been clearly demonstrated in many special instances in the United States, with prepaid health plans in turn offering a particularly attractive organizing principle for delivery of such services. However, these and related developments are unlikely to flourish and become generally available to the elderly citizens of the country as long as national health policy-making remains preoccupied with simply seeking private sector initiatives in quest of cutting costs within the country's current ill-conceived, fragmented system of health services. Rather, the critical next step is government-initiated fundamental structural reform toward achieving an integrated national health program.

While a strong political consensus for such fundamental reform of the nation's health care delivery system does not presently exist,* nonetheless for the first time in over a decade, various initiatives for a comprehensive national health policy have recently been promulgated. A number of these initiatives have come from constituencies particularly concerned with health care needs of the elderly. These initiatives include a proposal entitled "National Health Program for the United States," prepared by a coalition of national leaders in the American Public Health Association, including members of its gerontological health section (Terris 1984); a movement to establish a national health service, which counts among its strongest proponents the National Gray Panthers (1986), a senior-citizen-initiated social reform organization, and which received overwhelming approval in the form of a statewide referendum in the general election in Massachusetts in 1986 (personal communication, Authur Mazur, November 1986); the Harvard Medicare Project (1986) proposal for reforming and expanding the Medicare program (see ch. 10); and most recently, the U.S.Health Act of 1986 (H.R. 5070), introduced by California congressman Edward Roybal (1986), chairman of the House of Representatives Select Committee on Aging. All of these proposals include the following essential principles of a national health program: (1) universal enrollment of the population; (2) a single consolidated budget for personal health services; (3) comprehensive coverage, including preventive, acute, and chronic care; and (4) prepayment as a desirable form of reimbursement. The important

---

*Such a political movement may, however, be in the offing according to the following recent statement by Eli Ginsberg, (1985), a leading health economist and health policy adviser in the United States: "It is not farfetched to suggest that as more and more of the public become increasingly disgruntled by the mounting difficulties, congressmen looking for a way out would favor a dramatic new solution such as national health insurance or some variant" (p. 280). Furthermore, following the 1986 national elections which resulted in a Democratic Party majority in the Senate as well as in the House of Representatives, it has been suggested that a movement for a national health program is likely to become a leading political issue as the 1988 national elections approach ("The Great Debate" symposium featuring health policy staff members from the House and Senate, Annual Meeting of the Gerontological Society of America, November 21, 1986).

Finally and most currently, President Reagan's public endorsement of "catastrophic" health insurance for the elderly, in February 1987, while narrowly focused on high-cost hospitalizations, has provided a propitious opportunity for legislators to debate and deliver a comprehensive health care system (see Appendix M).

fiscal questions of how to finance the program and how to reimburse providers might be answered in a variety of traditional or nontraditional ways suggested in the various proposals that have been listed. A number of parties concerned with these issues, including the authors of the Roybal bill, recommend the model exemplified by the Canadian comprehensive health care system which combines the fiscal mechanism of government-operated universal health insurance with a mixture of prospective and fee-for-service reimbursement mechanisms. Once such essential enabling national policy for financing universal, comprehensive health services is in place, the way will truly be open for "the great energy and inventiveness of American medicine" to meet the challenges of providing appropriate services for its elderly. Without such system reform the chances seem poor.

APPENDIX A

Survey Instruments

Dear Dr

   We have become interested in factors which influence the decision to embark upon a career in Geriatric Medicine. After talking to quite a number of young consultants and senior registrars in the specialty, it has become apparent that there are many factors involved and we would like to attempt to identify which of these seem to be most important. It was considered that a useful exercise would be to seek information on these and related matters from doctors who have recently become consultants in Geriatric Medicine (or in General Medicine with special interest in Geriatric Medicine). We are therefore taking the opportunity of writing to all who became consultants during the period 1st January, 1978 and 31st December, 1982.

   Dr. William H Barker, a visiting Fellow in this Department from Rochester, New York, is involved in this study. He would also hope to carry out a parallel study in his own country when he returns this summer, and I think the comparison might be very interesting and revealing.

   We have devised a questionnaire which we believe is simple and easy to complete and will not take up much of your valuable time. I would be most grateful if you could complete the enclosed questionnaire and return it to me at your earliest convenience in the stamped, addressed envelope provided. I appreciate how irksome it can be to fill in yet another form, but I think you will probably agree that this might give us useful and much needed information on an important topic.

   We shall, of course, be happy to send you a summary of our findings when the survey is completed.

                                        Yours sincerely,

                                        J. WILLIAMSON

177

GERIATRIC CONSULTANT SURVEY QUESTIONNAIRE

1. NAME _____   2. Age in yrs. ____   3. ☐ Male ☐ Female

4. What post do you presently hold?
    ☐ Consultant in Geriatric Medicine
    ☐ Consultant Physician with Special Responsibility for Elderly
    ☐ Other _____

4a) Is your post an honorary (academic) NHS consultantship? ☐ Yes ☐ No

5. What year were you appointed to this post? _____

5a) At the time you were appointed, was the post
    ☐ A vacancy created by retirement, resignation or death?
       or
    ☐ A newly-created post?

6. What medical school did you attend for your undergraduate clinical medical course?
    _____

7. Year of qualification as a doctor _____

8. While you were a medical student did you have formal teaching in Geriatric Medicine?
    ☐ Yes   ☐ No
    If Yes, how would you best describe your teaching in Geriatric Medicine?
    ☐ Primarily clinical attachment
    ☐ Primarily theoretical activities (lectures, seminars, etc.)
    ☐ Other (please specify) _____
    _____

9. Please list your postgraduate qualification(s), using abbreviations (e.g. MRCP),
    and year obtained
             Qualification   Year obtained
             _____   _____

             _____   _____

             _____   _____

10. Have you taken a course in management of geriatric services?
    ☐ Yes   ☐ No   If Yes, tick (✓) which of the following:
                                  ☐ King's Fund Course
                                  ☐ Manchester Course
                                  ☐ Other _____

11. From the following list please tick (✓) the three most important factors
    in your decision to pursue a career in Geriatric Medicine.   Among these
    three, if there is one most important factor, please circle this one

    --- Positive experience in geriatrics in medical school

    --- Positive experience in geriatrics during postgraduate training

    --- Poor career prospects in specialty of first choice

    --- Preference for working with wide range of medical problems

    --- Opportunities for research

    --- Multi-disciplinary nature of the specialty

    --- Good opportunities for obtaining a consultant post

    --- Societal need for more physicians to care for the elderly

    --- Fitting in with family circumstances

    --- Career with community as well as hospital aspects

    --- Opportunities for teaching

    Other factors:

    _____

    _____

12. Did any one person, as a role model or counsellor, particularly influence you
    in making this decision? ☐ Yes ☐ No

    If Yes, please give his/her name and position (e.g. geriatrician,
    career counsellor, colleague)

    _____   _____
              Name   Position

    Comment (if you wish) _____

    _____

13. Please list in order below all posts which you have held since medical qualification,
    including locums of two months or longer.   For each post, please write in the space
    provided Specialty and Number of Years or Months in the post, and place a tick (✓)
    in the fourth column if the post included one month or more rotation in a Geriatric
    service.
    (Use common abbreviations; please print)

Post	Specialty	Time in post yrs., mos.	Geriatric rotation?	If Yes, No. mos.

14. At what stage did you first decide to pursue a career in Geriatric Medicine?

    _____   Which year? 19____

15. What other specialties did you seriously consider? Tick (✓) up to three
    from the following list:

    ☐ General Practice   ☐ Paediatrics   ☐ Rehabilitation

    ☐ General Surgery   ☐ General Medicine   ☐ Community Medicine

    ☐ Ob/Gyn.   ☐ Medical subspecialty: ☐ Other:

    ☐ Psychiatry   (specify) _____   (specify) _____

16. Was Geriatric Medicine your first preference?   ☐ Yes   ☐ No

    If No, which was your first preference _____

17. How well would you say your postgraduate training prepared you for your current
    responsibilities in Geriatrics?

    ☐ Very well   ☐ Moderately well   ☐ Poorly

    What, if any, clinical or non-clinical areas would you like to have learned more
    about before taking the post?   (list briefly)

    _____

    _____

    _____

18. In what, if any, ways would you like to change or improve your present unit?

    _____

    _____

    _____

19. If counselling medical students or house officers, what reasons would you give
    in favour of their pursuing a career in Geriatric Medicine?

    _____

    _____

    _____

    _____

    _____

Appendixes

181

Questions 20 - 31 deal with selected professional activities in the unit in which you currently work.

20. Are the unit's primary admission beds based in a teaching or district general hospital? ☐ Yes ☐ No

21. Which one of the following (a, b or c) best describes your unit?

a) ☐ Geriatric unit, admitting all or most medical patients above a certain age

If Yes, what is the cut-off age? _____

b) ☐ Geriatric unit, admitting patients selectively referred to geriatric medicine:

If Yes, are the majority of patients:

☐ Referred directly from the community

☐ Transferred from medical or surgical services

☐ Roughly equal number community admissions and transfers

c) ☐ Geriatric and general medicine unit, admitting adult medical patients of all ages

22. Do you furnish G.Ps in your area with written guidelines for referring patients to the unit? ☐ Yes ☐ No

(If Yes, please send a copy with return of this questionnaire, if one available. Thank you)

23. Approximately how many domiciliary or home assessment visits do you make a week? _____

24. Please tick (✓) Yes or No for each of the following statements.

Does the unit:

a) have one central coordinating office for keeping track of referrals, admissions, discharges, waiting list, etc. ☐ Yes ☐ No

b) routinely collect and compile statistics on number of referrals, admissions, discharges, domiciliary visits, etc. ☐ Yes ☐ No

c) regularly schedule holiday or respite ☐ Yes ☐ No

d) conduct a multi-disciplinary case conference one or more times a week ☐ Yes ☐ No

If Yes, tick (✓) disciplines regularly represented at these:

☐ Hospital Nursing ☐ Community Nursing ☐ Social Work

☐ Physiotherapy ☐ Occupational Therapy ☐ Speech Therapy

☐ Others (specify)

25. Does the unit have regularly scheduled liaison activities with the following services? (Tick ✓ if yes):

☐ General Medicine ☐ Orthopaedics

☐ Psychiatry ☐ Other _____

26. Is "bed-blocking" by elderly patients in acute units currently occurring as an important problem in your community? (i.e. are 5-10% of acute medical or surgical beds occupied by patients awaiting placement in a longstay hospital or residential accommodation?) ☐ Yes ☐ No ☐ Don't know

27. Tick (✔) Yes for each of the following patient care activities that are part of your regular weekly work; if possible, estimate number of sessions or half-sessions per week

Activity	Yes	No. Sessions
Assess. & Rehab. Ward		
Longstay Ward		
Outpatient Clinic		

28. Do you serve on any standing committees related to your work in geriatrics?

Tick (✔) any that apply

☐ In your hospital

☐ In your community or region

☐ National or International

29. Do you have regularly scheduled teaching responsibilities with any of the following? (Tick all that apply)

☐ Medical students   ☐ House officers   ☐ G.Ps

☐ Nurses   ☐ O.T. or P.T.   ☐ Others _____

30. During the past five years, have you been an active participant in any research projects related to geriatrics?

☐ Yes   ☐ No

If Yes, tick (✔) type(s) of research:

☐ Laboratory   ☐ Clinical   ☐ Epidemiological   ☐ Health Service

☐ Other (specify) _____

31. Have you been an author or co-author of any published papers (or to be published papers) related to geriatrics in the past 5 years?

☐ Yes   ☐ No

If Yes, tick (✔) the type of topic dealt with in the paper(s):

☐ Laboratory   ☐ Clinical   ☐ Epidemiological   ☐ Health Service

☐ Other (specify) _____

To   Doctors on the Lothian Health Board Medical List

From   William H. Barker, M.D. (on leave from Department of Preventive and Family
                                   Medicine, University of Rochester, New York)

Dear Dr.

    I am visiting in Edinburgh to study the provision of health and medical services
to the elderly.   The work of general practitioners in this regard is of particular
interest to myself and colleagues at home.   With the agreement of the General
Practitioners Subcommittee to the Lothian Area Medical Committee, I have accordingly
developed the following brief set of questions to address to GPs in the Lothian area.

    I would like to ask of you the favor of taking a few minutes to answer these
questions and return to me using the enclosed, pre-stamped and addressed envelope.

    As I wish to summarize this information before leaving at the end of June, I
would greatly appreciate your responding at your earliest convenience.   A summary
of my findings will be provided to you.

    Many thanks for your interest.

                            Sincerely yours,

---

1. PRACTICE

a) FOR HOW MANY YEARS HAVE YOU BEEN IN GENERAL PRACTICE? _____

b) WHICH OF THE FOLLOWING BEST DESCRIBES YOUR PRESENT PRACTICE ARRANGEMENTS?

   [ ] SINGLE-HANDED   [ ] PARTNERSHIP   [ ] HEALTH CENTRE

                          Number partners ____   Number GPs at Centre ____

c) WHICH OF THE FOLLOWING ARE ATTACHED TO THE PRACTICE ON A FULL-TIME OR PART-TIME
   BASIS?   (TICK ANY THAT APPLY)

   [ ] PRACTICE NURSE(S)   [ ] SOCIAL WORKER   [ ] PHYSIO.

   [ ] HEALTH VISITOR(S)   [ ] CHIROPODIST   [ ] O.T.

   [ ] DISTRICT NURSE(S)   [ ] PSYCHOLOGIST

---

2. ESTIMATES OF CERTAIN PATIENT CARE ACTIVITIES

a) PLEASE ESTIMATE THE NUMBER OF HOUSE CALLS YOU
   MAKE TO ELDERLY PATIENTS ON YOUR PRACTICE LIST   [ ] NONE   [ ] 1-2   [ ] 3-5
   ON AVERAGE IN A WEEK'S TIME.
   TICK (✔) BEST ESTIMATE.   [ ] 6-10   [ ] Greater than 10

b) PLEASE ESTIMATE THE NUMBER OF PATIENTS WHOM
   YOU REFER TO A GERIATRICIAN FOR ASSESSMENT   [ ] NONE   [ ] 1-2   [ ] 3-5
   OR CONSULTATION IN A YEAR'S TIME.
                                                      [ ] 6-10   [ ] Greater than 10
c) PLEASE ESTIMATE THE NUMBER OF PATIENTS ON
   YOUR PRACTICE LIST THAT ARE RESIDING IN   [ ] NONE   [ ] 1-5   [ ] 6-10
   NURSING HOMES OR OLD PEOPLE'S HOMES AT
   THE PRESENT TIME.   [ ] 11-25   [ ] 26-50

                                                      [ ] Greater than 50

3. SELECTED SERVICES RELATED TO ELDERLY WITHIN YOUR PRACTICE

  a) DO YOU KEEP AN AGE-SEX REGISTER IN YOUR PRACTICE?   Yes ☐ No ☐

  b) DO YOU HAVE A SYSTEM FOR ROUTINE MEDICAL SURVEILLANCE OF
     AN IDENTIFIED GROUP OF ELDERLY PATIENTS ON YOUR LIST?   Yes ☐ No ☐

  c) DO EITHER HEALTH VISITOR(S) OR DISTRICT NURSE(S) ATTACHED
     TO THE PRACTICE ROUTINELY VISIT AN IDENTIFIED GROUP OF
     ELDERLY PATIENTS ON YOUR PRACTICE LIST?   Yes ☐ No ☐

  d) DO YOU USE A STANDARD QUESTIONNAIRE OR SCALE FOR TESTING
     MENTAL STATUS IN ELDERLY PATIENTS?   Yes ☐ No ☐

  e) DO YOU ROUTINELY OFFER ANNUAL INFLUENZA VACCINATION TO AN
     IDENTIFIED GROUP OF "HIGH RISK" ELDERLY PATIENTS ON YOUR
     LIST?   Yes ☐ No ☐

4. INVOLVEMENT IN SERVICES TO ELDERLY OUTWITH YOUR PRACTICE LIST

   AMONG THE FOLLOWING SPECIAL SERVICES FOR THE ELDERLY, PLEASE TICK ANY ONE(S)
   FOR WHICH YOU CONTRACT TO PROVIDE ONE OR MORE SESSIONS PER WEEK

                                                       No. Sessions
                                                         per week

   ☐ GERIATRIC HOSPITAL   _____

   ☐ GERIATRIC DAY HOSPITAL   _____

   ☐ PSYCHOGERIATRIC HOSPITAL   _____

   ☐ PSYCHOGERIATRIC DAY HOSPITAL   _____

   ☐ PART IV OLD PEOPLE'S HOME(S)   _____

   ☐ VOLUNTARY OLD PEOPLE'S HOME(S)   _____

   ☐ PRIVATE NURSING HOME(S)   _____

   ☐ OTHER _____   _____

   _____   _____

   COMMENT, IF YOU WISH, ON THE MOST COMMON PATIENT PROBLEMS YOU ENCOUNTER IN
   PROVIDING THESE SERVICES.

5. PROFESSIONAL EDUCATION RELATED TO CARE OF THE ELDERLY

  a) HAVE YOU HAD FORMAL COURSEWORK OR TRAINING IN GERIATRICS DURING THE FOLLOWING
     STAGES OF YOUR CAREER?   PLEASE MAKE A TICK (✔) FOR ANY THAT APPLY.

     ☐ MEDICAL SCHOOL   ☐ GRADUATE TRAINING   ☐ POSTGRADUATE TRAINING

  b) PLEASE USE THE SPACE BELOW TO LIST CLINICAL OR NON-CLINICAL TOPICS RELATED TO
     CARE OF THE ELDERLY WHICH YOU WOULD RECOMMEND FOR INCLUSION IN POSTGRADUATE
     COURSES OR LECTURES FOR GPs.

   _____   _____

   _____   _____

   _____   _____

Please return this form in the enclosed pre-addressed envelope.
Thank you very much.

APPENDIX B

British Geriatrics Society
Memorandum on Provision of Geriatric Services, 1982

These recommendations are based either on official recommendations, published data, or a majority view approved by the BGS Council, November 19, 1981. It is emphasised that recommended facilities are based on minimum and not necessarily on optimum standards. Local situations and policies may demand weighing factors to reflect different patterns of service compatible with urban/rural practice, housing standards, family support available, and so forth. High turnover services require higher provision of resources. Recommendations relate to populations aged 65 and over having the average national age and sex structure, because services for the elderly have "statutory" responsibilities for that age group. It must be borne in mind however that the needs of the elderly increase exponentially throughout old age and differences or changes in the age distribution of local populations may have a disproportionate effect upon the need for provision.

Facilities for psychogeriatric care and the young disabled should not be included in the provision for geriatric services.

Hospital Geriatric Services

Within England and Wales we recommend that the hospital geriatric service should provide:

1. A minimum of 10 beds per 1,000 population aged 65 and over.
2. A minimum of 5 beds per 1,000 should be in the district general hospital or its equivalent.
3. Day hospital facilities of 1.5 to 2.0 places per 1,000 population aged 65 and over; at least half of these places to be in the district general hospital.
4. Out-patient facilities with X-ray and ready access to ECG and laboratory investigations.

Staff for Hospital-Based Geriatric Service

1. *Nursing Staff.* A minimum nurse/patient ratio of 1 to 1.16 (this recommendation has been adjusted for the 37½ hour working week of nursing staff) with a majority of trained staff.

185

2. *Rehabilitation Facilities:*
   a) *Physiotherapists*—five trained plus 5 helpers per 200 beds. Two trained plus 2 helpers per 40 day hospital places.
   b) *Occupational Therapists*—five trained plus 5 helpers per 200 beds. Two trained and 2 helpers per 40 day hospital places.
   c) *Social Workers*—hospital-based and 4 trained per 200 beds plus 1.5 trained for 40 day hospital places.
   d) *Speech Therapists*—two per 200 beds plus 40 day hospital places.
   e) *Dieticians*—one per 200 beds plus 40 day hospital places.
   f) *Dental Services*—five (half-day) sessions per week to service 200 beds and 40 day hospital places.
   g) *Chiropodists*—six (half-day) sessions per week per 200 beds and 40 day hospital places.
   h) *Health Visitors/Liaison Community Nurse*—two per 200 beds plus 40 day hospital places.
   i) *Audiometry*—one session per week per 200 beds plus 40 day hospital places.
   j) Availability of *optician* services on the hospital site.
   k) Orthotic services available.
   l) Hospital *voluntary services coordinator.*

Medical Staff

1. *Consultants.* Single-handed physicians responsible for geriatric medical services are not desirable and each district should have a minimum of two. No consultant should be expected to provide a service for more than seventy beds and twenty day hospital places. Consultant appointments may be entirely in geriatric medicine or have sessions in general medicine as well, but the two types of appointment should not be mixed within a single district. Teaching commitments require an increased number of consultants.

2. *Supporting Staff.* For district general hospital acute beds at least one pre-registration house officer, one SHO and one half registrar per nursing unit of twenty-four beds. For non-acute beds, these requirements may be halved. Multiple hospital sites may require an increase in SHO/HO staffing levels. All junior medical staff below senior registrar status must rotate into general medicine units to ensure adequate general professional training.

3. *Senior registrars* in approved training units.

4. *Administration for the Hospital-based Geriatric Service.* The administration should be centralised and include one higher clerical officer, two personal secretaries, one filing clerk per 200 beds. Additional secretarial assistance of at least one whole-time equivalent will be required for a day hospital of forty places and more if the day hospitals are separate. A ward clerk should be available on each ward.

APPENDIX C

Excerpt from Annual Report of NHS Hospital Advisory Service, 1973

A "Better Than Average" Service

Among the wide range of units visited were a number providing a very high standard of practice, which included a few of the well-known departments of geriatric medicine. Some units could be regarded as models in certain aspects of care, for example, in acute, rehabilitation or long-term care, but all units providing a better than average service had most of the following features:

1. At least one-third and sometimes one-half or more of the total allocation of geriatric beds were in a district hospital with full pathological, X-ray and other services available to them.
2. The remaining beds were usually in peripheral units. The total number of beds in most departments correspond with the national norm of 10 per 1,000 population over 65 years, but were sometimes either a little below or a little above this.
3. Although buildings were seldom new, there had been some imaginative upgrading. Wards were not overcrowded and had been provided with adequate privacy for patients and had easier access to a sufficient number of toilets.
4. The equipment was of good standard, there being a high proportion of adjustable height beds, a variety of chairs of differing heights suitable for old people, and modern aids for nursing which were being used.
5. More attention had been given to the content of the patients' day. Few cot sides and restricting chairs were in use. There was more participation of staff with patients in physiotherapy; and the incontinence rate was relatively low.
6. Practices such as "intermittent admission," holiday relief and progressive patient care were followed, the latter ensuring that the patient was in an environment most suited to his needs; there were separate areas for the alert and for the confused.
7. Great emphasis was laid on multidisciplinary management, the clinical team including the other staff being consulted in matters which affect ward management, e.g., purchase of equipment. There is no doubt that involving the staff in multidisciplinary management is of immense val-

187

ue to each member; it brings out new ideas, provides more job satisfaction and improves the image of and attitudes to geriatrics, thereby being an ultimate benefit to the patient.

8. The geriatric department had usually made a commitment to provide a comprehensive inpatient and outpatient service, accepting the care of all patients referred to them by general practitioners on an age-related basis (65+ or 75+), thus admitting urgent patients direct to the unit so that the department was able to deal with their problems from the start. This provides a more effective use of beds than allowing a patient to linger in an acute medical ward awaiting transfer to the geriatric wards.

9. A significantly high proportion of outpatients was seen in the better units. Clinics were held either at the hospitals, in the day hospital, or in health centres, and sometimes in all three. At least one clinic daily was held by the more progressive and active units. This emphasis on outpatient services is an important feature of units achieving a higher turnover of patients than average. It ensures that beds are always available for patients who need them, and where sufficient outpatient services existed, and this includes those seen at day hospitals, the waiting list was minimal.

10. Regular cases conferences involving the multidisciplinary clinical team also ensured a better use of resources. In some units these conferences are held weekly in the rehabilitation wards and on all patients after the first month of their admission, to reassess their progress. The case conferences are attended by members of the community health and social services teams and, in some instances, general practitioners and relatives may be invited to participate. A number of units have a health visitor or community nurses attached who are also fully involved in all matters concerning patient management.

11. Good relationships and communications existed between consultants in geriatrics and orthopaedic surgeons, as well as with psychiatrists and other colleagues.

12. There was also good collaboration with local authority social services and the community physician and his team, as well as with voluntary bodies.

13. It is usual to find that the administrative staff of the hospital have favourable attitudes towards the geriatric department.

14. It is significant too that the geriatric department had a better than average establishment of clerical and secretarial help, which not only maintained communication with general practitioners and local authorities, but also provided statistical information for the multidisciplinary team to enable them to monitor unit activity and provide a profile of ward performance. These are valuable incentives towards improving care.

15. A most significant aspect of units providing a good service was their higher-than-average establishment of medical staff: as well as more than one consultant geriatrician, these units frequently had junior staff in training grades, such as registrars and general practitioners' train-

ees. The nursing establishment was about level with the department's norm. The remedial staff may be few, but better use was made in these units of all resources, within both the hospitals and the community.

16. Very important is the maximum participation of trained social workers before the patient's admission, or immediately after, in sorting out problems from the start, so that help can be offered to the family as quickly as possible. In this way integration and resettlement into the community is far more successful than in areas where family difficulties are not often properly understood until the patient is discharged, when it is often too late.

17. Social workers made domiciliary visits so that the whole picture was available. Domiciliary visits were also made by consultants to prevent inappropriate admissions. Emphasis was rightly laid on patients returning to the community at the earliest stage compatible with medical and social competence.

18. Most of these units had an active training programme in geriatrics for their staff, but regrettably, owing to lack of facilities and time, were unable to undertake research.

Joint Statement by the Association of Directors of Social Services and the British Geriatrics Society

Medical Assessment for Elderly People Prior to a Move to Residential Accommodation

1. Research into the medical screening of elderly people accepted for residential care suggests that a significant proportion of such clients have treatable medical conditions and that appropriate treatment can improve the elderly person's condition to the extent that admission to residential care is unnecessary. Where a geriatric appraisal has been routinely carried out as part of a multidisciplinary approach to assessment, medical needs have been identified and more soundly based judgements made about the care required by the elderly person concerned.

2. There are many pressures on geriatric and psychiatric services but we feel that an input from these services when admission to residential care is under consideration could represent a good use of these resources because—

   a) Admission to residential care represents a point of crisis in the life of a client, often precipitated by physical and/or mental illness.

   b) Residential care is an expensive and scarce resource that should only be used by clients who need it.

   c) Admission itself may lead to an increased state of physical and/or psychological dependency.

   d) Admission in association with physical and mental dependency may be inappropriate if a remedial condition is present.

3. Whilst the final decision to admit a person to a local authority residential home will always rest with that authority or the applicant, we agree that medical assessment is desirable when admission is under consideration in order to ensure that—

   a) Medical problems are reviewed and appropriate treatment offered.

   b) Medical advice is available to the social services department so that the assessment of need is genuinely multidisciplinary.

   c) Full consideration is given to the possibility of alternative means of care—in a hospital, nursing home, sheltered housing or very sheltered housing, and to consider what support services would be required if the client were to remain in his/her own home.

d) Advice is available to staff of the home about the nature and level of the care required.

4. A medical assessment should be made by a doctor with special experience in geriatric medicine or the psychiatry of old age. Ideally, this should be before admission but we recognize that admission may take place in an emergency which may preclude such arrangements. In these situations we believe that medical assessment should take place within the first fourteen days of admission. To this end, and indeed to ensure that a complete social assessment is also available, all emergency admissions should be arranged on a short-term basis until assessment is complete. All medical assessments should be made in consultation with a patient's general practitioner. Patients from general hospital beds should be seen by a geriatrician, and sometimes a psychiatrist, before admission is effected.

5. The above arrangements represent good professional practice and if generally put into effect would secure a better use of medical and social services resources.

6. In many health districts and local authorities these arrangements could be implemented without additional resources.

7. We urge our respective members (in health districts and local authorities) to hold joint discussions at local level to review existing collaborative arrangements as to how these medical examinations should be instituted and to consider what changes are necessary to implement the recommendations of this joint statement.

8. The need for multidisciplinary assessment is equally applicable to people considering admission to private and voluntary residential care and nursing homes.

Topics for Discussion and Observation during Visits to Geriatrics Units on WHO-Sponsored Travel/Study Fellowship

1. *Origin and evolution* of the unit, particularly with respect to obtaining beds in district general or teaching hospital.
2. *Current structure and staffing,* including size of catchment population; number and location of beds; day hospital places; professional staff.
3. *Basic operations* of unit, as follows:
   a) *Admission policy,* e.g., source and criteria for admission, role of preadmission geriatric assessment.
   b) *Routine management,* e.g., central coordinating office for beds, arranging for holiday or respite admissions, multidisciplinary case conferences in assessment, rehabilitation and long-stay wards.
   c) *Day hospital,* e.g., degree to which this is used for long-term supportive care versus short-term assessment and rehabilitation.
4. *Consultant liaison activities* with other service sectors:
   a) General practitioners, e.g., any written guidelines for how and when to use geriatric consulting service.
   b) Other hospital services, e.g., general medicine, psychiatry, orthopedics, etc.
   c) Local authority social services, e.g., geriatric assessment of persons referred to residential accommodation.
   d) Local housing authority.
5. Status of following in the community served by the unit:
   a) "Bed blocking" in medical and surgical services.
   b) Availability of local authority residential accommodation (places per 1,000 over age 65).
   c) Psychogeriatric services.
   d) Transportation services, e.g., for day hospital.
   e) Availability of private nursing homes.
6. *Some broad general questions:*
   a) How does one best evaluate the impact of having geriatrics services as part of the NHS as opposed to not having these services?

b) What changes, improvements in geriatrics services, locally and/or nationally, are likely to occur in the next ten years?

7. *Academic activities* of the unit:
   a) *Teaching*—medical students, house officers, general practitioners, other health professionals.
   b) *Research*—basic, clinical, health services.

Medical Care in Great Yarmouth and Waveney Health District

In 1973 the geriatric services of the health district were led by two consultant geriatricians visiting from Norwich.* They looked after half the patients and a physician resident in the district looked after the other half (and also approximately half of the general medicine problems). The other half of the general medical problems were also managed by consultants visiting from Norwich. When the two geriatricians were about to be replaced, it was found impossible to recruit a whole-time geriatrician to the health district and the job was therefore readvertised for a general physician who would divide his time roughly 50 percent to geriatrics (which he would take over from the Norwich consultants) and 50 percent to general medicine. From February 1974, therefore, the General Medical and Geriatric services were run by two "integrated" general physician/geriatricians. The standard of SHO attracted to the geriatric post had previously been lower than for those we could attract to the general medical posts. In February 1976, therefore, we also integrated the junior staff to provide a unified service of four SHOs and one registrar. From that time all junior appointments were to the combined service.

The junior general medicine geriatric posts did not include a rotation since we wished to integrate patient care as well as hospital staffing. The admitting SHO was on call for all acute adult medical beds and admitted patients to wards by problem rather than by age. Recruitment of junior staff certainly improved and the various criteria of hospital bed usage (discharges and deaths, percentages bed occupation, average length of stay, turn-over interval) improved. We did not integrate ward care partly because of the "geriatric lead" for nurse salaries and partly because there was special nursing expertise on at least two of our wards. We appointed a third physician/geriatrician in 1978 and a fourth in 1981 and we intend to appoint a fifth in 1983. Two of these posts replaced existing consultants (nonintegrated) and one is a new post.

In the last two years there has been increasing criticism of the way the geriatric service has functioned. There are a number of identifiable reasons

*Provided by Dr. David Wayne, who originally prepared this description for use at a workshop held at the University of Manchester in 1982.

for this, many of them local and not relevant to discussion outside this health district. The most important criticism was, I think, about a lack of leadership when our unit expanded to four consultants with equal responsibilities. On September 1, 1982, we started a department of gerontology and appointed one of the four consultants as chairman. The post will be held for a year at a time by each of the four (or five) consultants in turn. The chairman will not only be responsible for problem-shooting but also will spearhead various initiatives for improving the service during his year of office. Another improvement to our services is the appointment of a senior registrar in geriatric medicine. He is expected to gain some experience of general medicine whilst spending two years with us and is rotating to Ipswich for the purely geriatric section of his experience and training.

We still feel that this integrationist approach to general medicine and geriatrics in our health district is the most appropriate at present. We have avoided the competition for resources between general medicine and geriatrics which occurs in other nonintegrated health districts and there is none of the personal antagonism which can be associated with this. We perform as many ward rounds on the acute admission geriatric wards as we do on the general medical wards. Since outpatients are fully integrated our figures according to age are not available: there is no difference in priority according to age.

Our arrangements, even without a rotating chairman, appear to have been effective in obtaining further facilities for the elderly of the health district, in that we have improved the standard of junior and middle-grade staffing, have created two day hospitals, much improved the rehabilitation services allocated for the elderly and will have doubled the number of available geriatric beds when the second phase of our hospital is opened in 1984. With the integration of the service many of the beds previously designated "general medicine" and not formally available for geriatric care became routinely used for medical problems of all kinds including the elderly.

The Spectrum of Care

J. Williamson

Figure A-1 shows, along the top half, the "spectrum of need" and, along the lower portion, the "continuum of care." The range and complexity of services increase progressively as we move from left to right. The fit elderly living in normal social settings require positive roles in family and society, together with preventive and primary care services of good quality. Then as social and medical problems increase, the effective coordination of services becomes more and more important, with the primary care health team playing a crucial role both as provider of services and as the instigator of other providers. Hence the whole system is dependent upon well-trained and well-motivated general practitioners and community nurses. As we move further along the chart the various specialist medical services become involved, as do residential accommodation and day-care facilities. At the far right lies the section of acute hospital care, and it is here that the results of imbalance of services become most apparent. Failure to provide adequate services in the preceding sections inevitably leads to inappropriate admission to the acute sector; even when the admission is "appropriate," there are likely to be delays in discharge because of blocked outflow channels. The lesson to be drawn from this simple diagram is that failure to provide any service in the continuum (or its provision in inadequate amount) will lead to a "domino" effect, with increased demand upon other services. "Bed blocking" within acute medical wards can thus never be solved by the mere provision of more residential and long-stay hospital resources—the only sure way is to ensure that the elements within the continuum of care are provided in the proper proportion and that they are effectively coordinated. This requires a good educational background for the providers of primary and secondary care, with a strong preventive emphasis and ready access to an efficient geriatric service.

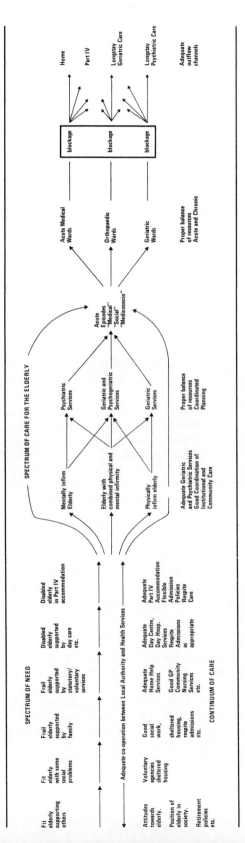

Figure A-1 The spectrum of care

Source: Williamson 1981.

Excerpts from Recommendations of the Commission on Chronic Illness

General Principles

Care of the chronically ill is inseparable from general medical care. While it presents certain special aspects, it cannot be medically isolated without running serious dangers of deterioration of quality of care and medical stagnation.

Care and prevention are inseparable: the basic approach to chronic disease must be preventive, and prevention is inherent in adequate care of long-term patients. Persons and institutions assuming care of the long-term patient have an obligation to apply early diagnosis and prompt and comprehensive treatment of the whole patient to prevent or postpone deteriorations and complications which may produce or aggravate disability.

Rehabilitation is an innate element of adequate care and properly begins with diagnosis. It is applicable alike to persons who may become employable and to those whose only realistic hope may be a higher level of self-care. Not only must formal rehabilitation services be supplied as needed, but programs, institutions, and personnel must be aggressively rehabilitation-minded.

Professional and administrative arrangements among institutions should be such as to facilitate easy transfer of patients from one to another in accordance with patient needs; and they should encourage the greatest possible continuity of care. Cooperative arrangements should extend to community health activities involved in providing care at home.

Community Care

Most long-term patients can best be cared for at home during much of their illness and prefer care in that setting under supervision of their personal physician. In spite of this, community planning continues to underemphasize such care. Comparatively little effort has been made to organize and provide the means whereby physicians can obtain for their patients the variety of services required to meet the diversified and complex needs that arise in long-term illness.

It is imperative that the patient's personal physician participate as continuously as possible in the medical care of each patient at all stages of illness. The physician determines the nature, time and place for the patient's diagnostic work-up and therapeutic services. The physicians, therefore, must equip themselves with knowledge of new methods of treating long-term illness; learn to use other health professions in care of the patient; and become familiar with community resources that offer the various services the patient may require.

In addition to physician services, long-term care for many patients— though by no means all—requires nursing, dental, social work, nutrition, homemaker, housekeeper, occupational therapy, physical therapy, and other rehabilitative services. In most communities these services, except nursing, are not yet available for the patient in his home. Communities are urged to make these services available and to develop methods to acquaint professional groups and the general public with them.

General Hospitals

The most desirable approach to providing hospital care to long-term patients is through extension, organization, and coordination of the facilities and services of general hospitals both private and public. In some general hospitals this will require only an extension of the hopsital's responsibility and reorientation of the staff so that diagnostic and therapeutic services—disproportionately dedicated to acute illness—will be appropriately and adequately applied to the chronically ill. In many other hospitals additional beds will be needed and personnel, space, and equipment required to provide specialized services to the long-term patient. In all general hospitals the concept, philosophy, and practice of rehabilitation must be paramount.

The independent chronic disease hospital is a second choice approach to long-term hospital care. It should be considered only when there is no practical way to associate the chronic disease facility physically and administratively with the general hospital. Where a special chronic disease hospital is unable to associate itself physically and organizationally with a general hospital, it must have adequate facilities and personnel for thorough diagnostic work-up, intensive study of the patient, and a dynamic program for definitive medical care and rehabilitation. The construction of new independent chronic disease hospitals (except research institutions) is not recommended.

Nursing Homes

Nursing homes and related institutions are essential for some phases of long-term illness. They are presently being operated under a variety of auspices— public; proprietary; and nonprofit voluntary such as religious and fraternal. Though there are many that are rendering excellent service, too many are operating unsatisfactorily.

Simultaneously and concurrently many of these institutions must yet equip themselves to provide safe and adequate care and become properly aligned with other community resources serving the chronically ill.

Individual physicians, medical societies, and hospital staffs particularly are urged to recognize the nature of the contribution which care in nursing and convalescent homes and homes for the aged can make and to help bring about necessary reforms.

On the basis of its studies and analysis of the problems, the commission believes that development of these institutions as elements of general hospitals is one of the best ways of raising standards, and recommends this arrangement. When outright affiliation is impossible, a close and active working relationship should be maintained.

Financing is probably the most neglected and unresolved area in improving care in the bulk of nonhospital institutions. The efforts of licensing authorities and nursing home operators to apply new knowledge and otherwise raise standards can succeed only if better financial support is forthcoming for these institutions, particularly the ones that are financed largely through public assistance. To provide a sounder financial basis for nonhospital institutions and the improvement of their standards, the commission recommends that:

a. Private insurance and prepaid medical and hospital plans extend the scope of benefits offered to include this type of service.

b. Responsible authorities make sufficient funds available to enable public agencies operating such facilities or purchasing this type of care to expend sufficient amounts to assure the quality of care required.

Education

Education for some classes of health personnel—particularly physicians and nurses—must be reoriented at undergraduate, graduate, and postgraduate levels. There is great need to balance instruction in the characteristics and treatment of short-term illness by placing equal emphasis on long-term illness. The characteristics of long-term illness require:

a. That the student gain full appreciation of the psychological and social factors that affect and are affected by long-term illness. In his training and experience, the student should see the patient in relation to his family and community, and should learn to use community resources in helping to meet the patient's economic, social, and spiritual needs.

b. That students have opportunities to observe and serve patients over a period sufficiently long to become fully aware of the changing nature of most long-term illness and to learn how to help the patient and his family through the various phases leading to maximum use of his capacities.

c. That there be training in the team approach to patient care. The curricula should include courses which emphasize the methods by which the various disciplines can and must work together in the care of long-term patients. Students in medicine, nursing, social work, physical therapy, occupational therapy, and other fields should have practical experience in jointly planning and carrying out patient care.

d. That students gain appreciation of the importance of continuity of care and the coordination of services to patients in their own homes, in nursing homes, in outpatient departments, and in rehabilitation centers.

e. That educational experience be offered in settings other than the hospital. Most long-term patients are cared for outside the hospital, yet most physicians and many other health personnel have their formal education in hospitals. Students should have experience in all the settings in which patients receive care, including their own homes.

Comparison of Benefits Covered under Medicare and Social Health Maintenance Organizations

Appendix I		
	Medicare Benefits	SHMO Benefits
Institutional services		
Acute hospital	90 days each benefit period plus 60-day lifetime reserve. $356 deductible per spell of illness on part A benefits required. Copays noted below are 1984 figures and assume deductible has been paid. For each day between days 61 and 90 the beneficiary pays $89. For each reserve day, the payment is $178.	Unlimited number of days for hospitalization at hospital approved by SHMO. Complete hospital services (inpatient and outpatient), including all physicians' and surgeons' services. No deductibles, no charges.
Psychiatric hospital	190 days lifetime. Copayments same as inpatient hospital.	190 days lifetime. No copays, no charges.
Skilled nursing facility care meeting Medicare criteria	After 3 consecutive days in hospital and then transferred to SNF: first 20 days no charge; days 21 thru 100: $44.50 per day.	No prior hospitalization requirement. No deductible, no charges. Kaiser and SCAN: 100 days. Elderplan: 365 days. Medicare Partners: unlimited days.
Skilled and intermediate nursing facility care of a custodial nature	Not covered.	Covered up to limits of chronic care benefit. Kaiser: 100 days, Elderplan: $6,500. Medicare Partners: $6,250. SCAN: $7,500. Coinsurance and benefit periods vary.

	Medicare Benefits	SHMO Benefits
Medical and related services Physician's services	Medicare pays 80% of allowable charges after $75 annual deductible on part B benefits is paid. Includes ambulatory (outpatient) surgery. Physicals and preventive care not covered.	Covers Medicare deductible and coinsurance. Ambulatory surgery, routine physician exam, preventive care included. Kaiser: $2 per visit. Elderplan includes authorized house calls by physician or physician extender.
Nurse practitioner and physician assistant services.	80% of allowable charges when provided incident to physician services.	Covered in full. Kaiser $2 per visit.
Mental health outpatient visits	80% of doctor charges up to $250 maximum (after $75 deductible). 80% of other professional charges.	Kaiser: 6 visits per year to psychiatrist; no limit to other professionals. Other sites: 20 visits per year. Copay per visit: Kaiser $2; Elderplan $5; Medicare Partners $10; SCAN no charges.
Foot care	Routine foot care services not covered except when performed as necessary part of a covered medical service. Medicare pays 80% of allowable charges.	Medically necessary podiatry. Kaiser $2 copay, other sites no charges. Elderplan in addition provides routine foot care at $2 per visit.
Blood	First 3 pints not covered; then 80% of allowable.	Covered in full.
Medical equipment and supplies	80% of allowable charges on durable medical equipment, prosthetic devices, and supplies.	Durable medical equipment, prosthetic devices and supplies covered in full when ordered and provided by plan.
Lab and X-ray	Part B services: 80% of allowable charges.	Covered in full.
Dentistry	80% of allowable charges only if it involves surgery of the jaw, setting fractures of the jaw and facial bones, treatment of oral infection, dental procedures that are integral part of medical procedures. Routine dental services not covered.	Medicare benefits covered in full—no charges. In addition, all sites cover dentures under the chronic care benefit limits, with copays (Kaiser 10%; Medicare Partners 20%; Elderplan and SCAN $50). SCAN also covers routine care; Medicare Partners covers diagnosis and preventive care; Elderplan covers erupted tooth extractions and denture repair ($15 copay).

(continued)

Appendix I (*Continued*)

	Medicare Benefits	SHMO Benefits
Outpatient physical therapy and speech pathology services	Part B services: 80% of allowable charges.	Medicare outpatient physical therapy speech pathology services covered in full by sites. No charges except Kaiser $2 regular fee.
Out-of-plan services	Emergency and non-emergency services covered anywhere in the United States.	Approved emergency services covered anywhere in the world. Kaiser and SCAN: no charges. Elderplan and Medicare Partners: 80% coverage of first $500, then same coverage as hospital and medical services described above.
Pharmacy	Not covered.	Prescription drugs covered at all sites. Copay range $1 to $3.50
Optometry	Only covered if related to treatment of aphakia or if part of a covered medical service.	Covered in full. Kaiser $2 copay. Elderplan specifies one exam per year.
Audiometry	Not covered.	Covered in full. Elderplan and Medicare Partners specify one exam per year. Kaiser $2 copay.
Eyeglasses	Not covered (contact lenses for postcataract surgery patients: approximately 80/20 per part B).	Covers one pair glasses in each 2–4 month period. Kaiser and SCAN: no charge. Elderplan $10 copay; Medicare Partners 50 percent copay.
Hearing aids	Not covered.	Covers one hearing aid in each 2–4 month period. Kaiser no charge. Copays: Elderplan $40; SCAN $50; Medicare Partners 50%.
Home health and other community-based services		
Medicare home health services (includes visiting nurse, home health aide; occupational, speech, and physical therapies, and social work services)	100% of allowable costs, skilled care criteria and homebound.	Medicare home health covered in full. Coverage expanded beyond skilled care and homebound criteria when approved for long-term care plan.
In-home support services (includes homemaker, personal health aide, medical transportation, medical day treatment, respite care and arranging and	Not covered.	Covered with limits, copays and renewability conditions (varies by site).

Medicare Benefits	SHMO Benefits

coordination of other services such as home-deliv-
ered meals, chore services,
additional transportation,
electronic monitoring)

Hospice (includes home health care, inpatient treatment for acute and chronic symptom control, family respite, outpatient drugs, counseling and volunteer services for terminal cancer patients)	5% copay or $5 per prescription for outpatient drugs, whichever is less. 5% copay for inpatient respite costs, up to a maximum of $304. All other hospice services are fully covered.	Covered in full (no copays).

Source: Leutz et al. 1985.

Services to be Included in Robert Wood Johnson Hospital Initiatives in Long-Term Care

Under this program, grantee hospitals are expected to:

1. Make available, in addition to existing acute care hospitals services, the following core of nontraditional services central to long-term care systems (providing at least two directly, and contracting for or providing directly the balance):
   — in-home health care services such as nursing and health aide services;
   — homemaker or home-help services, such as nutrition counseling, chore services, and transportation;
   — community-based mental health services for the elderly;
   — adult day care and/or day hospital services;
   — congregate or supported housing and/or sheltered residential care;
   — nursing home (skilled or intermediate); and
   — training and support for families and other care givers.

2. Serve, through its medical staff, as primary care providers for individuals without personal physicians.

3. Coordinate long-term care services with personal physicians of elderly individuals.

4. Provide directly all of the following supportive services:
   — case finding;
   — patient assessment, placement, monitoring, and follow-up;
   — quality assurance programs both for contracted and hospital-provided services;
   — 24-hour emergency services seven days a week;
   —centralized medical and service record and data systems; and
   —leadership in community long-term care planning.

(From Robert Wood Johnson Foundation Program for Hospital Initiatives in Long-Term Care, 1985)

"Preparation in Undergraduate Medical Education for Improved Geriatric Care"

Excerpt from Recommendations of the Executive Council of the Association of American Medical Colleges

Medical Management

Just as infants and children are not young adults, the elderly are not older middle-aged people. For this reason, the management of illnesses in older people differ from the management of the same illnesses in people of other ages. The following should be considered in development of the management plan.

Insofar as appropriate, independence and self-care should be encouraged.

The same preventive and therapeutic interventions are used for acute illness as for younger individuals with modifications based upon decreased functional capacity and the presence of chronic diseases in older patients.

Patients often have multiple chronic diseases; energetic treatment of one disease may affect another and may severely challenge the patient's diminished reserve of functional capacity.

For many patients, the therapeutic goal should be to slow progression of a disease or to diminish its disabling consequences rather than attempt a rapid cure. Small contributions can reduce disability and dependency.

Hazards for hospitalized elderly patients include nighttime confusion, falls, inapparent fractures, decubitus ulcers, fecal impaction, urinary retention, and prolonged convalescence.

The contributions of physical therapy, occupational therapy, and the other rehabilitation techniques to the improvement of functional capacity and capability for self-care should be recognized.

The physician should identify means to assist the patient in accommodating or preventing the loss of function and increase in disability brought about by specific diseases or the aging process.

Physicians should direct patients in an early stage of diseases leading to unpreventable deafness or blindness to special services provided by various agencies to prepare them in advance for these conditions.

The various health care and social service agencies providing comprehensive care should establish a constructive relationship.

Resources available in the community should be used to provide health care and social support, whether in the patient's own home, in a long-term care institution, or in other settings.

Family interrelationships may change over time as aging proceeds in the patient and in those providing care or as the care of the patient becomes more demanding.

Ethical and value issues often play a prominent and difficult part in decisions made about the care of elderly patients: (a) Determination of competency is of vital importance; the outcome of that determination may involve conflict between the best interests of the patient and those of the family, institution, or state. (b) Judgments surrounding the discontinuance of life-support systems can be enormously difficult and require consideration of the patient and the famliy as well as medical and legal factors.

Social and behavioral factors controlling health risks, environmental stressors, and health attitudes and behaviors are susceptible to interventive strategies and modifications. For example: (a) Certain existing old age disabilities can be reversed or alleviated. The performance of older people on intelligence tests improves with added practice, with instructions about strategies for approaching the problem, and with incentives to increase motivation and attention. (b) Older people can and often do learn to compensate for declines in reaction time, memory, and other age-related deficits. (c) Even in nursing homes, helpless, dependent, and unhappy patients can often recover a degree of functional independence when daily regimens encourage interaction, self-care, and a sense of mastery. Routines which stimulate independent behavior can result not only in increased alertness and involvement but also in improvements in general health.

(From *Journal of Medical Education* 1983. Supplement: Preparation in undergraduate medical education for improved geriatric care. Volume 58:501–27)

Recommendations for Health Service Development and Evaluation

Despite major differences both in ownership of health services (state-owned and operated in Great Britain; predominantly private ownership with public regulation in the United States) and in method of physician reimbursement (contracted salary in the former versus fee-for-service or prepayment with risk sharing in the latter), nonetheless, strategies and tactics evolved in Great Britain for providing comprehensive health care to the elderly appear to have exportable qualities that transcend ownership and reimbursement differences. Accordingly, the following recommendations, drawn from the British experience, are offered to academicians, clinicians, administrators, and health policy makers concerned with development and evaluation of innovative approaches to providing health services to the elderly in the United States.

A. *Delivery System*

Development of model health services that fiscally and professionally link primary medical care, acute and rehabilitative hospital care, and long-term care services, with the goal of minimizing unnecessary morbidity, maximizing independent functioning, and minimizing unnecessary use of acute or long-stay beds by elderly persons. Elements of such services, which call for special attention to both reimbursement policy and education of physicians and other involved health professionals, include:

1. *Primary Care.* Simple, valid techniques for identifying and monitoring at-risk elderly persons living in the community should be implemented along with tactics for responding promptly to alterations in such patients' health status, which might needlessly lead to hospital admission. The role of prompt home assessments of such patients by physicians or geriatric nurse practitioners should be considered and evaluated.

2. *Hospital Care.* Preferably the rehabilitation phase of care for elderly patients in acute hospitals with such needs would be initiated within the same department or hospital to which the patient is first admitted rather than after transfer to a separate rehabilitation facility or home health program, where discontinuity and lack of full knowledge of the

patient may significantly delay patient progress. Particular attention should be directed toward developing such broadened rehabilitation-oriented inpatient services for the elderly in general medical and selected surgical services (e.g., orthopedics) which are most likely to admit vulnerable elderly persons.

To guide development of these services, research on existing patient data from acute hospitals and skilled nursing facilities would be helpful in defining the amount and type of rehabilitation services (physical therapy, occupational therapy, speech therapy, social services, etc.) that might be required within a known population of elderly persons.

3. *Long-Term Care.* Those persons in need of continuing care who have family or other informal support in their own home should be provided sufficient formal support services to enable them to continue living in the community. As an adjunct to current "case management" strategies toward this end in the United States, day hospitals and planned respite admissions, two highly valued components of British geriatric services, designed to support the patient and his or her family, respectively, should be developed and evaluated.

Admissions to nursing homes should be largely limited to those patients unable to attain sufficient independence through hospital rehabilitation or community support services to live in their own homes. Medical care for intercurrent illness in nursing home residents should largely be provided within the facility, hence avoiding traumatic and costly transfer to acute hospitals whenever possible. Incentives for nursing homes and attending physicians to implement such acute services should be developed and their impact upon hospitalization evaluated.

B. *Personnel*

Career tracks should be developed for physicians, nurses, social workers, and members of the various remedial therapy professionals to acquire special expertise and assume explicitly designated roles in working with the problems of vulnerable elderly patients. Such training and positions would best be located primarily in the general hospital and nursing home sectors where the greatest concentration of patient needs for geriatric expertise will be encountered. The work patterns of such professionals would include multidisciplinary approaches to inpatient care as well as consultative linkages with patients' primary care physicians and community-based social, nursing, etc., support services.

C. *Data Monitoring*

Special studies and community surveillance systems should be developed to collect data with which to describe and quantitate health problems of elderly persons, and to describe and assess the extent to which personnel and organized services appropriate to meet these needs are being developed. Some priority areas in this regard include:

1. *Morbidity and Disability.* Data linking the occurrence of disability and dependency with identifiable medical morbidities. This will allow more discriminating predictions of how much rehabilitative and/or

long-term care may be expected to emerge from a given incidence of certain medical conditions, alone or in combination. The potential for prevention or early medical intervention to limit a portion of such disability and dependency may in turn be estimated and acted upon. (Such data, while available to some extent for stroke and hip fracture, are lacking for the vast majority of other chronic conditions of importance in old age.)

2. *Hospital-based Services.* Surveys of evolving efforts, largely by community hospitals, to "vertically integrate" primary care, inpatient acute and rehabilitative care, and both community-based and institutional long-term care. Information is needed on how such systems evolve from existing hospital operations to new forms of financing and integrating levels of care, and on how these organizational models impact on rates of acute and long-term institutionalization and overall cost of care for elderly persons whom they serve.

3. *Personnel.* Surveys of geriatric training programs and trainees to identify the special ingredients of such training as well as correctable gaps, to ascertain the types of career positions being assumed by graduates of this training, and to assess how well this effort is meeting the needs for geriatrics services in the country.

Comment on Catastrophic
Health Insurance Initiative

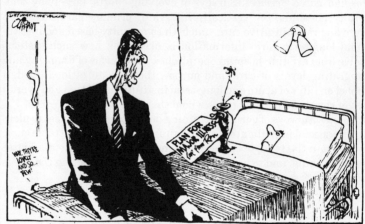

'WELL, I MUST BE RUNNING ALONG — ENJOY THE FLOWERS!'

Health care debate, at last

THE FEB. 13 article hailing President Reagan's "catastrophic" health insurance initiative is good news.

The good news, however, is not on page one, but on the inside (page 5A) where we learn that discerning members of the Senate and House are restless and wary of the "timid" nature of the catastrophic initiative (seems a paradox?).

The real ploy or paradox, politics if you will, is soon to follow (one may hope) as debate over a limited and ill-conceived catastrophic health insurance opens the legislative halls to a long overdue debate and delivery on a comprehensive health plan for the elderly. Such a plan must address the rehabilitation and long-term home care and nursing-home care that can play such a large part in the lives of older people.

This is a story in the making that all of us should watch and encourage.

William H. Barker, M.D.
Rochester

Barker is associate professor and consultant in health services, Monroe Community Hospital.

Source: Reprinted from Rochester *Democrat and Chronicle*, March 5, 1987, page 11A. Cartoon copyright 1987, Universal Press Syndicate. Reprinted with permission. All rights reserved.

References

Aaron, H. J., and Schwartz, W. B. 1984. *The painful prescription: Rationing hospital care*. Washington, D.C.: Brookings Institution.

Abel-Smith, B. 1964. *The hospitals, 1800–1848*. London: Heinemann.

Adams, G. F. 1961. Dr. Marjory Warren, C.B.E., 1897–1960. *Gerontologica Clinica* 3:1–4.

———. 1964. Clinical undertaking. *Lancet* 1:1055–58.

———. 1975. Eld health: Orgins and destiny of British geriatrics. *Age and Ageing* 4:65–68.

Aiken, L. H.; Mezey, M. D.; and Lynaugh, J. E., et al. 1985. Teaching nursing homes: Prospects for improving long-term care. *Journal of American Geriatrics Society* 33:196–201.

Allen, I. 1983. *Short-stay residential care for the elderly*. London: Policy Studies Institute.

American Association of Retired Persons. (AARP). 1984. Long term care research study. Washington, D.C.: AARP.

American College of Physicians. 1980. Proceedings of the Conference on the Changing Needs of Nursing Home Care. Philadelphia, Pa.

———. Health and Public Policy Committee. 1984. Long-term care of the elderly. *Annals of Internal Medicine* 100:760–63.

———. Health and Public Policy Committee. 1986. Home health care. *Annals of Internal Medicine* 105:454–60.

American Health Care Association. 1986. Hospitals and nursing homes: A new dialogue. *American Health Care Association Journal* 12:3–24 (special issue).

American Hospital Association. 1962. Background statement on role of hospitals in long-term care. American Hospital Association, Chicago,

Anderson, G. F., and Steinberg, E. P. 1984. Hospital readmissions in the Medicare population. *New England Journal of Medicine* 311:1349–53.

Anderson, W. F. 1974. Preventive aspects of geriatric medicine. *Journal of American Geriatrics Society* 22:385–92.

———. 1976. How geriatric medicine is being taught at the University of Glasgow. *Geriatrics,* 102–10.

Anderson, W. F., and Cowan, N. R. 1955. A consultative health centre for older people: The Rutherglen experiment. *Lancet,* 239–40.

Applegate, W. B.; Akins, D.; Vander Zwagg, R.; Thoni, K.; and Barker, M. G.

1983. A geriatric rehabilitation and assessment unit in a community hospital. *Journal of the American Geriatrics Society* 31:206–10.

Arcand, M., and Williamson, J. 1981. An evaluation of home visiting of patients by physicians in geriatric medicine. *British Medical Journal* 2:718–20.

Archer, R. L. 1970. Medicare and extended care facilities. *Hospitals* 44:48–51.

Arie, T. 1983. Teaching health care of the elderly in the medical course in Nottingham. *Age and Ageing* 12 (supp.):19–23.

Armstrong, D. 1983. *Political anatomy of the body: Medical knowledge in Britain in the twentieth century.* Cambridge: Cambridge University Press.

Ashley, J. S. A.; Laurence, D. J.; and Hughes, J. 1981. Inappropriate use of hospital beds: A survey of local investigations into the "blocked bed" problem. Department of Community Health, London School of Hygiene and Tropical Medicine. Typescript.

Bagnall, W. E.; Datta, S. R.; Knox, J.; and Horrocks, P. 1977. Geriatric medicine at Hull: A comprehensive service. *British Medical Journal* 2:102–4.

Barber, J. H., and Wallis, J. B. 1978. The benefits to an elderly population of continuing geriatric assessment. *Journal of the Royal College of General Practitioners* 28:428–33.

———. 1982. The effects of a system of geriatric screening and assessment on general practice workload. *Health Bulletin* 40:125–32.

Barber, J. H.; Wallis, J. B.; and McKeating, E. 1980. A postal-screening questionnaire in preventive geriatric care. *Journal of the Royal College of General Practitioners* 30:49–51.

Barker, L. F. 1943. Foreword. In *Geriatric medicine,* ed. E. J. Steiglitz. Philadelphia: W. B. Saunders.

Barker, W. H. 1984. An annotated list of readings and related resources on geriatric health services in Great Britain. *Journal of American Geriatrics Society* 32:623–27.

———. 1985. Development of innovative health services for the frail elderly: A comparison of programs in Edinburgh, Scotland and Rochester, New York. *Home Health Services Quarterly* 5:67–88.

———. 1986a. Case study of SeniorCare: A risk-based Medicare-HMO program. Typescript.

———. 1986b. Hospital-based geriatric services in Great Britain: Implications for the United States. *Pan American Health Organization Bulletin* 20:1–23.

Barker, W. H.; Williams, T. F.; Zimmer, J. G.; VanBuren, C.; Vincent, S.; and Pickrel, S. G. 1985. Geriatric consultation teams in acute hospitals: Impact on back-up of elderly patients. *Journal of the American Geriatrics Society* 33:422–28.

Barker, W. H., and Williamson, J. 1986. A survey of recently appointed consultants in geriatric medicine. *British Medical Journal* 293:896–99.

Beeson, P. B. 1985. The Institute of Medicine report in aging and medical education: 1984 update. *Bulletin of New York Academy of Medicine* 61:478–83.

Berg, R. L.; Browning, F. E.; Hill, J. G.; and Wenkert, W. 1970. Assessing the health care needs of the aged. *Health Services Research* 5:36–59.

Binks, F. A. 1968. Approach to disability and breakdown. *British Medical Journal* 1:269–74.

Blumenthal, D.; Schlesinger, M.; and Drumheller, P. B., et al. 1986. The future of Medicare. *New England Journal of Medicine* 314:722–28.

Bonano, J. B., and Wetle, T. 1984. HMO enrollment of Medicare recipients: An analysis of incentives and barriers. *Journal of Health Politics, Policy, and Law* 9:41–62.

Bonham-Carter, D. 1969. *Functions of the district general hospital.* Report prepared for the Department of Health and Social Security. London: Her Majesty's Stationery Office.

Boucher, C. A. 1957. *Survey of services to the chronic sick and elderly, 1954–1955.* Ministry of Health Reports on Health and Medical Subjects, no. 98. London: Her Majesty's Stationery Office.

Bowen, O. R., and Burke, T. R. 1985. Cost neutral catastrophic care proposed for Medicare recipients. *Federation of American Health Review* (Nov.–Dec.):42–45.

Boyd, R. V.; Hawthorne, J.; Wallace, W. A.; Worlock, P. H.; and Compton, E. H. 1984. The Nottingham orthogeriatric unit after 1000 admissions. *Injury* 15:193–96.

Boyd, W. D.; Woodside, M.; and Zealley, A. K. 1979. Psychogeriatric consultation: A review of 100 home and hospital visits in Edinburgh. *Health Trends* 37:202–7.

Boyer, N.; Chuang, J. C.; and Gipner, D. 1986. An acute care geriatric unit. *Nursing Management* 17:22–25.

Braverman, A. M. 1975. Geriatric patients in acute medical wards. *British Medical Journal* 4:703.

Brickner, P. W.; Duque, T.; and Kaufman, A., et al. 1975. The homebound aged: A medically unreached group. *Annals of Internal Medicine* 82:1–6.

British Geriatrics Society. 1982. Memorandum on provision of geriatric services. London.

British Geriatrics Society and Royal College of General Practitioners. 1978. Training general practitioners in geriatric medicine. *Journal of Royal College of General Practitioners* 28:355–59.

British Geriatrics Society and Royal College of Nursing Working Party. 1975. *Improving geriatric care in hospitals.* Royal College of Nursing, London.

British Medical Association. 1947. *The care and treatment of the elderly and infirm.* London.

———. 1965. *Charter for the family doctor service.* London.

———. 1976. *Care of the elderly.* London: British Medical Association.

Brocklehurst, J. C. 1984. Conference on vocational training in geriatric medicine. *Age and Ageing* 13:179–80.

———, ed. 1983. Teaching geriatric medicine to medical students. *Age and Ageing* 12, supp. 1.

Brocklehurst, J. C., and Andrews, K. 1985. Geriatric medicine: The style of practice. *Age and Ageing* 14:1–7.

Brocklehurst, J. C.; Leeming, J. T.; Carty, M. H.; and Robinson, J. M. 1978. Medical screening of old people accepted for residential care. *Lancet* 2:141–43.

Brocklehurst, J. C., and Tucker, J. S. 1980. *Progress in geriatric day care.* London: King Edward's Hospital Fund.

Brody, S. J. 1985. *Rehabilitation and nursing homes.* In *The teaching nursing home,* ed. E. L. Schneider et al., pp. 147–56. New York: Raven Press.

———. 1986. Impact of the formal support system on rehabilitation of the elderly. In *Aging and rehabilitation: Advances in the state of the art,* eds. S. J. Brody and G. E. Ruff, pp. 62–86. New York: Springer Publishing Company.

Brody, S. J., and Magel, J. S. 1984. DRG: The second revolution in health care for the elderly. *Journal of American Geriatrics Society* 32:676–79.

Brody, S. J., and Persily, N. A., eds. 1984. *Hospitals and the aged: The new old market.* Rockville, Md.: Aspen Systems Corporation.

Brook, E. B. 1948. The place of the out-patient department in caring for old people. *Medical Press* (May):400–402.

Brown, N. K., and Thompson, D. J. 1979. Nontreatment of fever in extended-care facilities. *New England Journal of Medicine* 300:1246–50.

Buckley, E. G. 1977. Personal points of view: The role of the general practitioner in the geriatric assessment unit. *Health Bulletin* 35:323–26.

Burley, L. E. 1983. The joint geriatric orthopaedic service in South Edinburgh. In *Advanced geriatric medicine 3,* ed. F. I. Caird and J. G. Evans, pp. 137–43. London: Pittman.

Burley, L. E.; Currie, C. T.; Smith, R. G.; and Williamson, J. 1979. Contribution from geriatric medicine within acute medical wards. *British Medical Journal* 2:90–92.

Burton, J. R. 1985. The house call: An important service for the frail elderly. *Journal of the American Geriatrics Society* 33:291–93.

Butler, R. N. 1981. The teaching nursing home. *Journal of the American Medical Association* 245:1435–37.

Campion, E. W. 1980. Personal view. *British Medical Journal* 281:1002.

Campion, E. W.; Bang, A.; and May, M. I. 1983. Why acute-care hospitals must undertake long-term care. *New England Journal of Medicine* 308:71–75.

Campion, E. W.; Jette, A.; and Berkman, B. 1983. An interdisciplinary geriatric consultation service: A controlled trial. *Journal of the American Geriatrics Society* 31:792–96.

Carboni, D. K. 1982. *Geriatric medicine in the United States and Great Britain.* Westport, Conn: Greenwood Press.

Career prospects in geriatrics. 1980. *British Medical Journal* 1:426.

Carroll, D. 1966. History of the Baltimore City Hospitals. *Maryland State Medical Journal* 15:2–6.

Coe, R. M.; Brehm, H. P.; and Peterson, W. A. 1974. Impact of Medicare on the organization of community health resources. *Health and Society* 62:230–65.

Coid, J., and Crome, P. 1986. Bed blocking in Bromley. *British Medical Journal* 292:1253–56.

Collard, A. F.; Bachman, S. S.; and Beatrice, D. F. 1985. Acute care delivery for the geriatric patient: An innovative approach. *Quality Review Bulletin* 11:180–85.

Commission on Chronic Illness. 1956. *Care of the long-term patient.* Vol. 2. Cambridge: Harvard University Press.

Conable, B. B. 1982. Medicare Long-Term Care Act of 1982. *Congressional Record,* 22 April 1982. Washington, D.C.: Government Printing Office.

Coni, N. K. 1975. Geriatric patients in acute medical wards. *British Medical Journal* 4:703.

Connolly, M. P. 1980. Health visiting, 1850–1900: A review. *Midwife, Health Visitor, and Community Nurse* 16:282–85.

Cosin, L. Z. 1955. The organization of a day hospital for psychiatric patients in a geriatric unit. *Proceedings of the Royal Society of Medicine* 49:237–39.

———. 1971. Testimony before Senate Subcommittee on Long-Term Care of the Special Committee on Aging. Pp. 1375–1419. Washington, D.C.: Government Printing Office.

Courtney, H. A. 1973. Personal points of view: The role of the general practitioner in a geriatric assessment unit. *Health Bulletin* 31:211–14.

Currie, C. T.; Burley, L. E.; and Doull, C., et al. 1980. A scheme of augmented home care for acutely and sub-acutely ill elderly patients: Report on pilot study. *Age and Ageing* 9:173–80.

Currie, C. T.; Moore, J. T.; Friedman, S. W.; and Warshaw, G. A. 1981. Assessment of elderly patients at home: A report of fifty cases. *Journal of the American Geriatrics Society* 29:398–401.

Currie, C. T.; Smith, R. E.; and Williamson, J. 1979. Medical and nursing needs of elderly patients admitted to acute medical beds. *Age and Ageing* 8:149–51.

Dalgaard, O. Z. 1982. Care of the elderly in Denmark: Special aspects including geriatric and long-term medicine. *Danish Medical Bulletin* 29:89–168.

Das Gupta, P. K. 1980. Developing an active geriatric service in Scunthorpe. *Public Health, London* 94:155–60.

Davies, B., and Challis, D. 1980. Experimenting with new roles in domiciliary social service: The Kent Community Care Project. *Gerontologist* 20:292–99.

Davis, K., and Rowland, D. 1986. *Medicare policy: New directions for health and long-term care.* Baltimore: Johns Hopkins University Press.

Day, P., and Klein, R. 1985. Central accountability and local decision making: Towards a new NHS. *British Medical Journal* 290:1676–78.

DeLargy, J. 1957. Six weeks in: Six weeks out. *Lancet* 1:418–19.

Devas, M. B. 1977. *Geriatric Orthopaedics.* London: Academic Press.

Donaldson, M. 1985. Career aspirations of geriatric medicine trainees. *Age and Ageing* 14:8–10.

Dunlop, B. D. 1976. Need for and utilization of long-term care among elderly Americans. *Journal of Chronic Disease* 29:75–87.

Dunn, A. M., and Patel, K. P. 1983. Integration of geriatric with general medical services. *Lancet* 2:1139.

Ealey, J., and Ealey, T. 1983. Payment fallout from Medicare. *Contemporary Administrator* (Sept.):33–35.

Eggert, G. M.; Bowlyow, J. E.; and Nichols, C. S. 1980. Gaining control of the long-term care system: First returns from the ACCESS experiment. *Gerontologist* 20(3):356–63.

Epstein, A.; Hall, J.; and Besdine, R., et al. 1985. Structure of ambulatory GAUs. *Gerontologist* 25:62.

Evans, J. G. 1981. Institutional care. In *Health of the elderly: Essays in old age medicine, psychiatry and services,* ed. T. Arie. London: Croom Helm.

———. 1983. Integration of geriatric with general medical services in Newcastle. *Lancet* 1:1430–33.

Evans, J. G., and Graham, J. M. 1984. Medical care of the elderly: Five years on. *Journal of the Royal College of Physicians of London* 18:18–20.

Evashwick, C. J.; Rundall, T.; and Goldiamond, B. 1985. Hospital services for older adults. *Gerontologist* 25:631–37.

Exton-Smith, N. 1952. Investigation of the aged sick in their homes. *British Medical Journal* 2:182–86.

Feder, J., and Scanlon, W. 1982. The underused benefit: Medicare's coverage of nursing home care. *Milbank Memorial Fund Quarterly* 60:604–32.

Feller, B. A. 1983. Americans needing help to function at home. National Center for Health Statistics. *Advancedata* 92:1–11.

Fisk, A. 1983. Comprehensive health care for the elderly. *Journal of American Medical Association* 249:230–36.

Forsyth, G., and Logan, F. L. 1964. Medical technology and the needs of chronic disease. *Journal of Chronic Disease* 17:789–802.

Frengley, J. D. 1985. History of geriatric program. Metropolitan General/Highland View Hospital, Cleveland. Typescript.

Freymann, J. G. 1980. *The American health care system: Its genesis and trajectory.* Huntington, N.Y.: Krieger Publishing.

Fries, B. E., and Cooney, L. M. 1983. A patient classification system for long-term care. Typescript.

Fries, J. F. 1980. Aging, natural death, and the compression of morbidity. *New England Journal of Medicine* 303:130–35.

Gale, J., and Lively, B. 1974. Attitudes towards geriatrics: A report of the King's survey. *Age and Ageing* 3:49–53.

Gatherer, A. A. 1981. Support in the home. Ch. 3 in *The impending crisis of old age,* ed. R. F. A. Shegog. Oxford: Oxford University Press.

General Medical Council Education Committee. 1980. *Recommendations on basic medical education.* London: General Medical Council.

Gibbins, F. J.; Lee, M.; Davison, P. R.; O'Sullivan, P.; Hutchison, M.; and Murphy, D. R. 1982. Augmented home nursing as an alternative to hospital care for chronic elderly invalids. *British Medical Journal* 284:330–33.

Gillick, M.; Serrell, N. A.; and Gillick, L. S. 1982. Adverse consequences of hospitalization in the elderly. *Social Science and Medicine* 16:1033–38.

Gillick, M., and Steel, K. 1983. Referral of patients from long-term to acute-care facilities. *Journal of American Geriatrics Society* 31:74–78.

Ginsberg, E. 1985. The restructuring of U.S. health care. *Inquiry* 22:272–81.

Godber, G. 1982. Striking the balance: Therapy, prevention, and social support. *World Health Forum* 3:258–75.

Gornick, M.; Greenberg, J. N.; Eggers, P. W.; and Dobson, A. 1985. Twenty years of Medicare and Medicaid: Covered populations, use of benefits, and program expenditures. *Health Care Financing Review* Annual Supplement:13–59.

Graham, J. M., and Playfair, H. R. 1983. General medicine with special responsibility for the elderly. *Health Trends* 15:66.

Gray Panthers. 1986. The critical condition of health care in the U.S. *Gray Panther Network*, Spring 1986. Entire issue devoted to reforming health care system.

Great Britain. Department of Health and Social Security. 1971. Hospital geriatric services. Administrative memorandum F/G54/71.

———. 1976. *Priorities for health and social services in England*. London: Her Majesty's Stationery Office.

———. 1979. Physicians in geriatric medicine and physicians with a special responsibility for the aged. Administrative memorandum B/M/169/2D.

———. 1981a. *Report of a study on community care*. London: DHSS Information Division.

———. 1981b. *The respective roles of the general acute and geriatric sectors in care of the elderly hospital patient*. London: DHSS Information Division.

———. 1983. *Elderly people in the community: Their service needs*. London: Her Majesty's Stationery Office.

———. Ministry of Health. 1962. *A hospital plan for England and Wales*. London: Her Majesty's Stationery Office.

———. National Health Service. 1946. Report of negotiating committee. *British Medical Journal* (supp.):123–27.

Green, M. 1975. Services for the elderly. In *Specialized futures: Essays in honor of Sir George Godber*, pp. 101–53. London: Oxford University Press.

Greenberg, J. N.; Leutz, W.; Ervin, S.; Greenlick, M.; Kodner, D.; and Selstad, J. 1985. S/HMO: The social/health maintenance organization and long term care. *Generations* (Summer):51–55.

Gritzer, G., and Arluke, A. 1985. *The making of rehabilitation: A political economy of medical specialization, 1890–1980*. Berkeley and Los Angeles: University of California Press.

Growing older. 1981. Cmnd. 8173. London: Her Majesty's Stationery Office.

Gruenberg, E. M. 1977. The failures of success. *Milbank Memorial Fund Quarterly* 55:3–24.

Grundy, E. 1983. Demography and old age. *Journal of American Geriatrics Society* 31:325–32.

Haber, C. 1983. *Beyond sixty-five: The dilemma of old age in America's past*. Cambridge: Cambridge University Press.

Harrington, C. 1985. Alternatives to nursing home care. *Generations* (Summer):43–46.

Harvard Medicare Project. 1986. *New England Journal of Medicine* 314:722–28.

Hay, E. H. 1976. A geriatric survey in general practice. *Practitioner* 216:443–47.

Hazzard, W. R. 1986. An American's ode to British geriatrics revisited. *Age and Ageing* 15:307–11.

Heinz, J. 1985. News. U.S. Senate Special Committee on Aging. 26 February 1985. Washington D.C.

Hildick-Smith, M. 1984. Geriatric day hospitals: Changing emphasis in costs. *Age and Ageing* 13:95–100.

Hilfiker, D. 1983. Allowing the debilitated to die: Facing our ethical choices. *New England Journal of Medicine* 308:716–19.

Hodkinson, H. M., and Jeffries, P. M. 1972. Making hospital geriatrics work. *British Medical Journal* 2:536–39.

Hollingsworth, J. R. 1986. *A political economy of medicine: Great Britain and the United States.* Baltimore: Johns Hopkins University Press.

Hospitals for chronic and incurable cases. 1896. *Boston Medical and Surgical Journal* 135:347–48.

Howell, T. 1974. Origins of the British Geriatrics Society. *Age and Ageing* 3:69–72.

Hughes, S. L. 1985. Apples and oranges? A review of evaluation of community-based long-term care. *Health Services Research* 20:461–88.

Hutt, R.; Parsons, D.; and Pearson, R. 1981. The timing and reasons for doctor's career decisions. *Health Trends* 13:17–20.

Iglehart, J. K. 1985. Medicare turns to HMOs. *New England Journal of Medicine* 312:132–36.

Ingman, S. R.; Lawson, I. R.; and Carboni, D. 1978. Medical direction in long-term care. *Journal of American Geriatrics Society* 26:157–66.

Institute of Medicine. 1978. *Aging and medical education.* Washington, D.C.: National Academy of Sciences.

———. 1986. *Improving the quality of care in nursing homes.* Washington, D.C.: National Academy Press.

Irvine, P. W.; VanBuren, N.; and Crossley, K. 1984. Causes for hospitalization of nursing home residents: The role of infection. *Journal of the American Geriatrics Society* 32:103–7.

Irvine, R. E. 1963. Progressive patient care in the geriatric unit. *Postgraduate Medical Journal* 39:401–7.

———. 1980. Geriatric day hospitals: Present trends. *Health Trends* 12:68–71.

Isaacs, B., and Evers, H., eds. 1984. *Innovations in the care of the elderly.* London: Croom Helm.

Isaacs, B.; Livingston, M.; and Neville, Y. 1972. *Survival of the unfittest.* London: Routledge and Kegan Paul.

Isaacs, B., and Thompson, J. 1960. Holiday admissions to a geriatric unit. *Lancet* 1:969–71.

Johnson, M., and Challis, D. 1983. The realities and potentials of community care. In *Elderly People in the Community: Their Service Needs.* London: Her Majesty's Stationery Office. Chapter 6, 93–117.

Johnson, C. L., and Grant, L. A. 1985. *The nursing home in American society.* Baltimore: Johns Hopkins University Press.

Johnson, T. E. 1985. Geriatrics and medical education: Initiatives of the

Association of American Medical Colleges. *Bulletin of the New York Academy of Medicine* 61:484–91.
Joint Commission on Higher Medical Training. 1980. Training handbook and third report. London: Royal College of Physicians.
Jolley, D.; Smith, P.; and Bellington, L., et al. 1982. Developing a psychogeriatric service. Ch. 10 in *Establishing a geriatrics service,* ed. C. Davis. London: Croom Helm.
Jones, D. A., and Vetter, N. J. 1985. Formal and informal support received by carers of elderly dependents. *British Medical Journal* 291:643–45.
Kane, R. L.; Jorgensen, L. A.; Teteberg, B.; and Kuwahara, J. 1976. Is good nursing home care feasible? *Journal of American Medical Association* 235:516–19.
Kane, R. L.; Solomon, D.; Beck, J.; Keller, E.; and Kane, R. 1980. The future need for geriatric manpower in the United States. *New England Journal of Medicine* 302:1327–32.
Katz, S.; Branch, L. G.; and Branson, M. H., et al. 1983. Active life expectancy. *New England Journal of Medicine* 309:1219–23.
Kavesh, W. N.; Mark, R. G.; and Kearney, B. 1984. Medical care teams improve nursing home care and reduce costs. Paper presented at Annual Meeting of Gerontological Society of America, November 1984.
Kayser-Jones, J. S. 1981. *Old, alone, and neglected: Care of the aged in Scotland and the United States.* Berkeley and Los Angeles: University of California Press.
———. 1982. Institutional structures: Catalysts of or barriers to quality care for the institutionalized aged in Scotland and the U.S. *Social Science and Medicine* 16:935–44.
Kennedy, R. D. 1984. The British National Health Service. *New England Journal of Medicine* 310:1672.
Klein, R. 1983. *The politics of the National Health Service.* London: Longman.
Knickman, J. R., and McCall, N. 1986. A prepaid managed approach to long-term care. *Health Affairs* 4:94–104.
Koren, M. J. 1986. Home care—Who cares? *New England Journal of Medicine* 314:917–20.
Kovar, M. G. 1983. The United States elderly people and their medical care. Background paper for Commonwealth Fund Forum 1983 on Improving the Health of the Homebound Elderly. London.
Lave, J. R. 1985. Cost containment policies in long-term care. *Inquiry* 22:7–23.
Lefton, E.; Bonstelle, S.; and Frengley, J. D. 1983. Success with an inpatient geriatric unit: A controlled study of outcome and followup. *Journal of American Geriatrics Society* 31:149–55.
Leonard, J. C. 1976. Can geriatrics survive? *British Medical Journal* 1:1335–36.
Leutz, W. 1986. Long-term care for the elderly: Public dreams and private realities. *Inquiry* 23:134–40.
Leutz, W. N.; Greenberg, J. N.; and Abrahams, R., et al. 1985. *Changing health care for an aging society.* Lexington, Mass.: D. C. Heath.

Levenson, S. A.; List, N. D.; and Zaw-Win, B. 1981. Ethical considerations in critical and terminal illness in the elderly. *Journal of the American Geriatrics Society* 29:563–67.

Liang, M. H.; Gall, V.; Partridge, A.; and Eaton, H. 1983. Management of functional disability in homebound patients. *Journal of Family Practice* 17:429–35.

Libow, L. S. 1982. Geriatric medicine and the nursing home: A mechanism for mutual excellence. *Gerontologist* 22:134–44.

Libow, L. S., and Cassel, C. K. 1985. Fellowships in geriatrics. *Bulletin of New York Academy of Medicine* 61:547–57.

Lichtenstein, H., and Winograd, C. H. 1984. Geriatric consultation: A functional approach. *Journal of the American Geriatrics Society* 32:356–61.

Liem, P. H.; Chernoff, R.; and Carter, W. J. 1986. Geriatric rehabilitation unit: A 3-year outcome evaluation. *Journal of Gerontology* 41:44–50.

Littauer, D.; Steinberg, F. U.; and Gee, G. A. 1963. A chronic disease unit in a general hospital: Analysis of six years' operating experience. Chicago: American Hospital Association.

Lowe, C. R., and McKeown, T. 1949. The care of the chronic sick. *British Journal of Social Medicine* 3:110–26.

Lowther, C. P.; MacLeod, R. D. M.; and Williamson, J. 1970. Evaluation of early diagnostic services for the elderly. *British Medical Journal* 2:275–76.

Lowther, C. P., and Williamson, J. 1966. Old people and their relatives. *Lancet* 2:1460.

Lubitz, J., and Deacon, R. 1982. The rise in the incidence of hospitalization for the aged, 1967 to 1979. *Health Care Financing Review* 3:21–40.

Luft, H. S. 1981. *Health maintenance organizations: Dimensions of performance.* New York: John Wiley and Sons.

Lye, M. 1982. Geriatric medicine and general unemployment. *Journal of the Royal College of Physicians of London* 16:129–31.

McAlpine, C. J. 1979. Unblocking beds: A geriatric unit's experience with transferred patients. *British Medical Journal* 2:646–48.

McArdle, C.; Wylie, J. C.; and Alexander, W. D. 1975. Geriatric patients in an acute medical ward. *British Medical Journal* 4:568–69.

McKeown, T. 1973. A conceptual background for research and development in medicine. *International Journal of Health Services* 3:17–28.

McKeown, T.; Mackintosh, J. M.; and Lowe, C. R. 1961. Influence of age on type of hospital to which patients are admitted. *Lancet* 1:818–20.

Maeda, N. 1985. Medical care costs for the aged in Japan. Paper presented at Thirteenth International Congress of Gerontology, New York, 14 July 1985.

Maklan, C. 1984. Geriatric specialization in the U.S.: Profile and prospects. Ph.D. diss., University of Michigan. University Microfilms International, Ann Arbor, Mich.

Mamber, M. 1980. Hospital backlog. *Medical World News* 63–70.

Manton, K. G. 1982. Changing concepts of morbidity and mortality in the elderly population. *Milbank Memorial Fund Quarterly* 60:183–244.

Marmor, T. R. 1970. *The politics of Medicare.* Chicago: Aldine.

Martin, D. C.; Morycz, R. K.; and McDowell, J., et al. 1985. Community-based geriatric assessment. *Journal of the American Geriatrics Society* 33:602–6.

Martinez, F. M.; Carpenter, A. J.; and Williamson, J. 1984. The dynamics of a geriatric day hospital. *Age and Ageing* 13:34–41.

Master, R. L.; Feltin, M.; and Jainchill, J., et al. 1980. A continuum of care for the inner city: Assessment of its benefits for Boston's elderly and high-risk populations. *New England Journal of Medicine* 302:1434–40.

Mather, H. G.; Morgan, D. C.; and Pearson, N. G., et al. 1976. Mycardial infarction: A comparison between home and hospital care for patients. *British Medical Journal* 1:925–29.

Mather, J. H., and Abel, R. W. 1986. Medical care of veterans: A brief history. *Journal of American Geriatrics Society* 34:757–60.

Mather, J. H., and Dube, W. F. 1981. Veterans Administration's development of health profession's education programs in geriatrics and gerontology. Ch. 23 in *The geriatric imperative,* ed. A. R. Somers and D. R. Fabian. New York: Appleton-Century-Crofts.

Matthews, D. A. 1984. Dr. Marjory Warren and the origin of British geriatrics. *Journal of American Geriatrics Society* 32:253–58.

Means, R., and Smith, R. 1985. *The development of welfare services for elderly people*. London: Croom Helm.

Mechanic, D. 1975. Ideology, medical technology, and health care organization in modern nations. *American Journal of Public Health* 65:241–47.

Meiners, M. 1983. The case for long-term care insurance. *Health Affairs* 2:55–79.

Millard, P. H., and Smith, C. S. 1981. Personal belongings: A positive effect. *Gerontologist* 21:85–90.

Miller, F. H., and Miller, G. A. H. 1986. *The painful prescription:* A procrustean perspective? *New England Journal of Medicine* 314:1383–86.

Milne, J. S. 1985. *Clinical effects of ageing: A longitudinal study*. London: Croom Helm.

Moore, J. T., and Fillenbaum, G. G. 1981. Change in functional disability of geriatric patients in a family medicine program: Implications for patient care. *Journal of Family Practice* 12:59–66.

Moore, J. T.; Warshaw, G. A.; and Walden, L. D., et al. 1984. Evolution of a geriatric evaluation clinic. *Journal of the American Geriatrics Society* 32:900–905.

Morishita, L.; Sui, A.; and Wang, R. et al. 1986. Geriatric day hospital: Innovative comprehensive hospital-based outpatient care. *Gerontologist* 26:242A.

Mott, P. D., and Barker, W. H. 1987. Hospital and medical care utilization by nursing home patients: The effect of patient care plans. *Journal of the American Geriatrics Society* (in press).

Mundinger, M. D. 1983. *Home care controversy: Too little, too late, too costly*. Rockville, Md.: Aspen Systems Corporation.

Murphy, F. W. 1977. Blocked beds. *British Medical Journal* 1:1395–96.

National Institute on Aging. 1983. Conference on assessment. *Journal of the American Geriatrics Society* 31:636–64, 721–65.

———. 1984. Report on education and training in geriatrics and gerontology. Typescript.

National Study Group on State Medicaid Strategies. 1983. Restructuring Medicaid: An agenda for change. Washington, D.C.: Center for Study of Social Policy.

Nepean-Gubbins, L. 1972. The home help service: Past, present, and future. *Community Health* 4:77–82.

New York Academy of Medicine. 1985. Symposium on the Geriatric Medical Education Imperative. *Bulletin of the New York Academy of Medicine,* vol. 61.

Norton, A. 1981. Collaboration to meet the needs of the elderly. In *The impending crisis of old age: A challenge to ingenuity,* ed. R. F. A. Shegog. London: Oxford University Press.

O'Brien, T. D.; Joshi, D. M.; and Warren, E. W. 1973. No apology for geriatrics. *British Medical Journal* 2:277–80.

The old woman with a broken hip. 1982. Editorial. *Lancet* 2:419–20.

Oriol, W. E. 1985. *The complex cube of long term care: The case for next step solutions—Now.* Washington, D.C.: American Health Planning Association.

Panneton, P. E.; Moritsugu, K. P.; and Miller, A. M. 1982. Training health professionals in care of the elderly. *Journal of American Geriatrics Society* 30:144–49.

Pastore, J. O.; Winston, F. B.; Barrett, H. S.; and Foote, F. M. 1968. Characteristics of patients and medical care in New Haven area nursing homes. *New England Journal of Medicine* 279:130–36.

Pater, J. E. 1981. *The making of the National Health Service.* London: King Edward's Hospital Fund.

Pathy, M. S. 1982. Operational policies. Ch. 3 in *Establishing a geriatric service,* ed. D. Coakley. London: Croom Helm.

Pathy, M. S.; Hughes, S. N. P.; and White, W. M. 1972. Role for the specialist health visitor in the geriatric team. *Community Medicine* 15:206–7.

Peach, H., and Pathy, M. S. 1982. Attitudes towards the care of the aged and to a career with elderly patients among students attached to a geriatric and general medical firm. *Age and Ageing* 11:196–202.

Pike, L. A. 1976. Screening the elderly in general practice. *Journal of the Royal College of General Practitioners* 26:698–703.

Primrose, W. R., and Capewell, A. E. 1986. A survey of registered nursing homes in Edinburgh. *Journal of the Royal College of General Practitioners* 36:125–28.

Private nursing homes. 1985. *Lancet* 2:1338–40.

The question of a hospital for chronic disease. 1906. *Boston Medical and Surgical Journal* 154:444–45.

Rae, J. W., Jr.; Smith, E. M.; and Lenzer, A. 1962. Results of a rehabilitation program for geriatric patients in a county hospital. *Journal of American Medical Association* 180:463–68.

Rafferty, J.; Smith, R. G.; and Williamson, J. 1987. Medical assessment of elderly persons prior to a move to residential care: A review of seven years experience in Edinburgh. *Age and Ageing* (in press).

Rai, G. S.; Murphy, P.; and Pluck, R. A. 1985. Who should provide hospital care of elderly people? *Lancet* 1:683–85.

Rango, N. 1982. Nursing home care in the United States: Prevailing conditions and policy implications. *New England Journal of Medicine* 307:883–89.

Reedy, B. 1979. The health team. In *Trends in general practice, 1979,* ed. J. Fry. London: British Medical Association.

Rice, D.P., and Feldman, J. J. 1983. Living longer in the United States: Demographic changes in health needs of the elderly. *Health and Society* 61:362–96.

Rich, B. M., and Baum, M. 1984. *The aging: A guide to public policy.* Pittsburgh: University of Pittsburgh Press.

Robbins, A.; Mather, J.; and Beck, J. 1982. Status of geriatric medicine in the United States. *Journal of American Geriatrics Society* 30:211–18.

Robert Wood Johnson Foundation. 1985. The foundation's program for hospital initiatives in long-term care: Presentation of planning grants for 25 sites. Princeton, N.J. Typescript.

Rodstein, M. 1979. Contributions of the long-term care facility to the medical care of the aged. *Journal of American Geriatrics Society* 27:410–13.

Rogers, D. E. 1983. Where does the geriatrician fit? *Journal of American Geriatrics Society* 31:124–25.

Royal College of Physicians of Edinburgh. 1963. *The care of the elderly in Scotland.* Publication No. 22.

———. 1970. *The care of the elderly in Scotland: A follow-up report.* Publication No. 37.

———. 1981. *Appropriate care for the elderly: Some problems.* Publication No. 54.

Royal College of Physicians of London. 1972. Report of the college committee on geriatric medicine.

———. 1977. Report of the working party on medical care of the elderly. *Lancet* 1:1092–95.

Roybal, E. 1986. News. U.S. House of Representatives Select Committee on Aging. June 23, 1986.

Rubenstein, L. Z.; Abrass, I. B.; and Kane, R. L. 1981. Improved geriatric care for patients on a new geriatric evaluation unit. *Journal of American Geriatrics Society* 29:531–36.

Rubenstein, L. Z.; Josephson, K. R.; Nichol-Seamans, M.; and Robbins, A. S. 1986. Comprehensive health screening of well elderly adults: An analysis of a community program. *Journal of Gerontology* 41:342–52.

Rubenstein, L. Z.; Josephson, K. R.; and Wieland, G. D., et al. 1984. Effectiveness of a geriatric evaluation unit: A randomized clinical trial. *New England Journal of Medicine* 311:1664–70.

Rubenstein, L. Z.; Rhee, L.; and Kane, R. L. 1982. The role of geriatric assessment units in caring for the elderly: An analytic review. *Journal of Gerontology* 37:513–21.

Rubenstein, L. Z.; Wieland, G. D.; Josephson, K. R.; Dunn, S.; and Sayer, J. 1985. Relative odds of institutionalization and death for frail elderly in-

patients and the impact of geriatric assessment and treatment. *Gerontologist* 25:62.

Rubin, S. G.; and Davies, G. H. 1975. Bed blocking by elderly patients in
general-hospital wards. *Age and Ageing* 4:142–47.

Ruchlin, H. S.; Morris, J. N.; and Eggert, G. M. 1982. Management and
financing of long-term-care services: A new approach to a chronic problem. *New England Journal of Medicine* 306:101–5.

Schler, S. H.; Erickson, R. V.; and Strickler, J. C. 1985. The aging of populations: Clinical care of the elderly. *Journal of American Geriatrics Society*
33:509.

Schlesinger, M. 1986. On the limits of expanding health care reform: Chronic
care in prepaid settings. *Milbank Quarterly* 64:189–215.

Schweinitz, K. 1961. *England's road to social security.* New York: A. S. Barnes
and Co.

Schweitzer, S. O., and Greenburg, E. R. 1984. Do social services reduce the
use of hospitals by the elderly. In *Promoting the well-being of the elderly,*
ed. M. F. Collen and and H. R. Oldfield. Symposium of the International
Health Evaluation Association, London.

Shanas, E. 1974. Health status of older people: Cross national implications.
American Journal of Public Health 64:261–64.

Shaughnessy, P. W., and Tynan, E. A. 1985. The use of swing beds in rural
hospitals. *Inquiry* 22:303–15.

Sheldon, J. H. 1948. *The social medicine of old age.* London: Oxford University Press.

———. 1971. A history of British geriatrics. *Modern Geriatrics* 457–64.

Schock, N. W.; Gruelich, R. C.; and Andres, R., et al. 1984. *Normal human
aging: The Baltimore longitudinal study of aging.* NIH Publication No.
84-2450. Bethesda, Md.

Silver, C. P. 1978. Patterns of delivery of care by departments of geriatric
medicine. Ch. 9 in *Recent advances in geriatric medicine,* vol. 1, ed. B.
Isaacs. Edinburgh: Churchill Livingstone.

Smith, R. G., and Williams, B. O. 1983. A survey of undergraduate teaching
of geriatric medicine in the British medical schools. *Age and Ageing* 12
(supp.):2–16.

Smits, H., and Draper, P. 1974. Care of the aged: An English lesson? *Annals
of Internal Medicine* 80:747–53.

Somers, A. R. 1976. Geriatric care in the United Kingdom: An American
perspective. *Annals of Internal Medicine* 84:466–76.

———. 1982. Long-term care for the elderly and disabled: A new health
priority. *New England Journal of Medicine* 307:221–26.

Somers, A. R., and Fabian, D. R. 1981. *The geriatric imperative.* New York:
Appleton-Century-Crofts.

Starr, P. 1982. *The social transformation of American medicine.* New York:
Basic Books.

Steel, K. 1984. Geriatric medicine is coming of age. *Gerontologist* 24:367–72.

———, ed. 1981. *Geriatric education.* Lexington, Mass: Collamore Press.

Steel, K., and Hays, A. 1981. A consultation service in geriatric medicine at a university hospital. *Journal of American Medical Association* 245:1410–11.

Stephen, P. J., and Williamson, J. 1984. Drug-induced parkinsonism in the elderly. *Lancet* 2:1082–83.

Stevens, R. 1966. *Medical practice in modern England*. London: Heinemann.

———. 1971. *American medicine and the public interest*. New Haven: Yale University Press.

———. 1977. Geriatric medicine in historical perspective: The pros and cons of geriatric medicine as a specialty. Paper presented at the National Institute on Aging, March 18.

Stout, R. W., ed. 1985. Teaching gerontology and geriatric medicine. *Age and Ageing* 14, supp. 1.

Suzman, R., and Riley, M. W., eds. 1985. The oldest old. *Milbank Memorial Fund Quarterly* 63:177–451. Special issue.

Teasdale, T. A.; Shuman, L.; Snow, E., and Luchi, R. 1983. A comparison of placement outcomes of geriatric cohorts receiving care in a geriatric assessment unit and on general medicine floors. *Journal of American Geriatrics Society* 31:529–34.

Terris, M. 1984. A national health program for the United States: The need for a citizen's coalition. *Journal of Public Health Policy* 5:10–17.

Thompson, A. P. 1949. Problems of aging and chronic sickness. *British Medical Journal* 22:243–50, 300–305.

Thompson, M. K. 1984. *The care of the elderly in general practice*. Edinburgh: Churchill Livingstone.

Thurlow, R. M. 1972. Extended Medicare: A new disappearing act. *Medical Economics* 186–202.

Tinker, A. 1981. *The elderly in modern society*. London: Longman.

de Tocqueville, A. [1848] 1958. Preface. In *Democracy in America*, trans. Phillip Bradley. Reprint. New York: Vintage Books.

Townsend, P. 1962. *The last refuge*. London: Routledge and Kegan Paul.

Townsend, P., and Wedderburn, D. 1964. *The aged in the welfare state*. London: Bell.

Tulloch, A. J., and Moore, V. 1979. A randomized controlled trial of geriatric screening and surveillance in general practice. *Journal of the Royal College of General Practitioners* 29:733–42.

U.S. Department of Commerce. Bureau of the Census. 1982. *1980 census and middle series estimates: Projection of the population of the United States. 1980–2050.* Current Population Reports, series P-25, no. 922. Washington, D.C.: Government Printing Office.

U.S. Department of Health and Human Services. Health Care Financing Administration. 1984. Medicare program: Prospective payment for Medicare inpatient services. Final rule. *Federal Register* 49:234–40.

———. National Center for Health Statistics. 1982. Changes in mortality among the elderly: United States, 1940–78. DHHS Publication No. (PHS) 82-1406. Washington, D.C.: Government Printing Office.

———. Office of the Inspector General. 1980. Restricted patient admittance to nursing homes: An assessment of hospital back up. Washington, D.C.

U.S. Department of Health, Education, and Welfare. National Center for Health Statistics. 1979. The national nursing home survey. DHEW Publication No. (PHS) 79-1794. Washington, D.C.: Government Printing Office.

VanBuren, C. B.; Barker, W. H.; Williams, T. F.; and Zimmer, J. G. 1982. Acute hospitalization of nursing home patients: Characteristics, costs, and potential preventability. *Gerontologist* 22:179.

Verbrugge, L. M. 1984. Longer life but worsening health? Trends in health and mortality of middleaged and older persons. *Health and Society* 62:475–519.

Vetter, N. J.; Jones, D. A.; and Victor, C. R. 1984. Effect of health visitors working with elderly patients in general practice: A randomized controlled trial. *British Medical Journal* 288:369–72.

Vladeck, B. C. 1980. *Unloving care: The nursing home tragedy.* New York: Basic Books.

Vladeck, B. C., and Firman, J. P. 1983. The aging of the population and health services. *Annals of the American Academy of Political Science* 468:132–48.

Vogel, R. J., and Palmer, H. C. 1985. *Long-term care: Perspectives from research and demonstrations.* Rockville, Md.: Aspen Systems.

Wan, T. H.; Weissert, W. G.; and Liveratos, B. B. 1980. Geriatric day care and homemaker services: An experimental study. *Journal of Gerontology* 35:256–74.

Ward, D. H. 1984. A nursing home management system for doing more for less: The responsive caregiving model. Paper commissioned for the National Academy of Sciences, Washington, D.C.

Warren, M. W. 1946. Care of the chronic aged sick. *Lancet* 1:841–43.

———. 1948. The evolution of a geriatric unit. *Geriatrics* 3:42–50.

Warshaw, G. A.; Moore, J. T.; and Friedman, S. W., et al. 1982. Functional disability in the hospitalized elderly. *Journal of American Medical Association* 248:847–50.

Wattis, J.; Wattis, L.; and Arie, T. 1981. Psychogeriatrics: A national survey of a new branch of psychiatry. *British Medical Journal* 2:1929–33.

Weissert, W. G. 1985. The cost-effectiveness trap. *Generations* (Summer):47–50.

Weissert, W. G.; Wan, T. H.; Liveratos, B. B.; and Pellegrino, J. 1980. Cost-effectiveness of homemaker services for the chronically ill. *Inquiry* 17:230–43.

Weksler, M. E.; Durmaskin, S. C.; and Kodner, D. L. 1983. New goals for education in geriatric medicine. *Annals of Internal Medicine* 99:856–57.

Wexler, R. 1986. The cost of cost control. *City Newspaper* 15:4.

Wieland, D.; Rubenstein, L. Z.; Ouslander, T. G.; and Martin, S. E. 1986. Organizing an academic nursing home: Impacts on institutionalized elderly. *Journal of the American Medical Association* 255:2622–27.

Wilcock, G. K.; Gray, J. A. M.; and Pritchard, P. M. M. 1982. *Geriatric problems in general practice.* New York: Oxford University Press.

Willard, H., and Kasl, S. V. 1972. *Continuing care in a community hospital.* Cambridge: Harvard University Press.

Williams, M. E., and Williams, T. F. 1986. Evaluation of older persons in the ambulatory setting. *Journal of the American Geriatrics Society* 34:37–43.

Williams, T. F. 1981. Clinical and service aspects of geriatric teaching programs. In *The geriatric imperative,* ed. A. R. Somers and D. R. Fabian. New York: Appleton-Century-Crofts.

———. 1985. The geriatric medical education imperative. *Bulletin of the New York Academy of Medicine* 61:471–77.

Williams, T. F.; Hill, J. G.; Fairbank, M. E.; and Knox, K. G. 1973. Appropriate placement of the chronically ill aged: A successful approach to evaluation. *Journal of the American Medical Association* 226:1332–35.

Williams, T. F.; Izzo, A. J.; and Steel, K. 1975. Innovations in teaching about chronic illness and aging in a chronic disease hospital. Ch. 3 in *Teaching of chronic illness and aging,* ed. D. W. Clark and T. F. Williams. DHEW Publication No. (NIH) 75-876. Bethesda, Md.: Fogarty International Center, National Institutes of Health.

Williamson, J. 1979. Geriatric medicine: Whose specialty? *Annals Internal Medicine* 91:774–77.

———. 1981. The spectrum of care. In *Appropriate care for the elderly: Some problems.* Publication No. 54. Royal College of Physicians of Edinburgh.

———. 1984. Health care of the elderly: Theory and practice. *Nova Scotia Medical Bulletin*:103–8.

———. 1987. Perspective from the United Kingdom. In *Reshaping health care for the elderly,* ed. C. Eisdorfer. Baltimore: Johns Hopkins University Press.

Williamson, J.; Burley, L. E.; and Smith, R. G. 1986. *Looking after old people in primary care.* Bristol: John Wright and Sons.

Williamson, J., and Chopin, J. M. 1980. Adverse reactions to prescribed drugs in the elderly: A multicentre investigation. *Age and Aging* 9:73–80.

Williamson, J.; Lowther, C. P.; and Gray, S. 1966. The use of health visitors in preventive geriatrics. *Gerontologica Clinica* 8:362–69.

Williamson, J.; Stokoe, I. H.; and Gray, S., et al. 1964. Old people at home: Their unreported needs. *Lancet* 1:1117–20.

Wolff, M. L.; Smolen, S.; and Ferrara, L. 1985. Treatment decisions in a skilled-nursing facility: Discordance with nurses preferences. *Journal of the American Geriatrics Society* 33:440–45.

Worden, G. L. 1985. Impact of a risk-based Medicare demonstration on a continuing care department. Paper presented at meeting of Group Health Association of America, June 1985.

World Health Organization. 1982. Teaching gerontology and geriatric medicine: Report on a workshop, Edinburgh, 5–7 April 1982. World Health Organization publication no. ICP/ADR 045(2).

Yordi, C. L., and Waldman, J. 1985. A consolidated model of long-term care: Service utilization and cost impacts. *Gerontologist* 25:389–97.

Zawadski, R. T., ed. 1983. *Community-based systems of long term care.* New York: Haworth Press.

Zawadski, R. T., and Ansak, M. L. 1983. Consolidating community-based long-term care: Early returns from the On Lok demonstration. *Gerontologist* 23:364–69.

Zimmer, J. G.; Brodows, B.; Treat, A.; and Eggert, G. M. 1987. Nursing homes as acute care providers: An experiment with financial incentives to reduce hospitalizations. *Journal of the American Geriatrics Society* (in press).

Zimmer, J. G.; Groth-Juncker, A.; and McCusker, J. 1985. A randomized controlled study of a home health care team. *American Journal of Public Health* 75:134–41.

Zwick, D. I. 1985. Home health services for the elderly: The English way. In *International perspectives of long term care,* ed. L. Reif and B. Trager. New York: Haworth Press.

Index

232   Index

Brocklehurst, J. C., 54, 100
Butler, R. N., 147

Canada: and comprehensive health
care, 175; and geriatric medicine,
171
Career, medical (G.B.): development of,
87–89; diagram of, 88
Care of the Elderly in Scotland (1963,
1972), 27
Case management, 86, 123, 126, 142–
45, 153–54, 163–64
Catastrophic health insurance, xv, 127,
174, 212
Catchment areas, geriatric services in,
25, 33–34, 48–49, 170
Center for Gerontological Research of
the U.S. Public Health Service, 146
Channeling projects, 142
Clinical Effects of Aging (1985), 45
Commission on Chronic Illness (U.S.,
1956), 109; recommendations, 198–
201
Community care: Great Britain, 11, 28,
73–86, 196–97; United States, 114–
16, 125–26, 139–46, 199. *See also*
General practice; Long-term care;
Nursing; Social services
Complex Cube of Long Term Care
(1985), 158
Comprehensive care for elderly: elements in Great Britain, 101–2, 170;
illustrations, 11, 24, 60, 157, 163,
196–97; initiatives in U.S., 154–64,
172–75; recommendations for development, 209–11, 212
Compression of morbidity thesis (1980),
3
Conable, B., bill in U.S. Congress, 126
Connecticut Triage Program, 141
Consultant, geriatric. *See* Geriatric
medicine
Consultation, geriatric, 40–43, 132–33;
ad hoc patterns in Great Britain,
55–56; joint services, 56; orthopedic
surgery, 41, 56, 59, 71; psychiatry,
42–43, 56–57; routine, 55–56; tactics, 58–59. *See also* Monroe County
Continuum of care. *See* Comprehensive
care for the elderly
Cosin, L.Z., 54, 108, 120–22

Cost containment (U.S.), 122–40, 159,
172–73
Custodial care, Medicare definition of,
113

Day hospital, 25, 37–40, 48–49, 54–55,
96, 151, 155
Death rate, for elderly (U.S., 1940–78),
3
Deficit Reduction Act (1984), 160
Delayed time of death model, 4
Denmark and geriatric medicine, 172
Department of Health and Social Se-
curity (DHSS) (G.B.), 25, 28
Diagnosis related group (DRG), 2, 130,
138; payment limitation, 145; *The
Second Revolution in Health Care for
the Elderly* (1984), 145. *See also*
Medicare
Disability of elderly, 4–9, 152
Discharge planning, 36–37, 52, 70, 132,
145, 159–63. *See also* Multidisciplin-
ary team
District general hospital (G.B.), 25–27
DRG. *See* Diagnosis related group

Ebenezer Society of Minneapolis, 161
Edinburgh, Scotland, and geriatrics:
augmented home care, 63–64; case
conference, multidisciplinary, 36–
37; City Hospital, 33–40; consultations, 40–43, 70–71; geriatric day
hospital, 38–40; geriatric inpatient
unit, 39; geriatric medicine units,
33–34; geriatric orthopedic rehabilitation unit (GORU), 41; health
professionals, 34–35; home visits,
37–38; Longmore Hospital, 33; long-
stay facility, 64–65; map of, 34; psychogeriatric services, 41–43; Royal
Edinburgh Hospital, 41; Royal Infirmary, 40, 41; Royal Victoria Hospital, 33; School of Primary Health
Care in the Elderly, 44; University
of Edinburgh, 33; university department of geriatric medicine, education, and research, 43–45. *See also*
Lothian Health Board
Elderly (U.S.), health status of: compression of morbidity thesis, 3;
death rate for 65 and older, 3; de-

ADDING LIFE TO YEARS

Designed by Ann Walston.

Composed by the Composing Room of Michigan, Inc.
in Century Schoolbook with ITC Century Bold Condensed display.

Printed by the Maple Press Company
on 50-lb. S.D. Warren Sebago Eggshell Cream offset
and bound in Holliston Roxite A cloth.